THE YOGA SCIENCE

A Complete Guide to Strength, Flexibility, and Injury Prevention

DIVYANSH SHARMA

HAY HOUSE

HAY HOUSE INDIA
New Delhi • London • Sydney
Carlsbad, California • New York City

Hay House Publishers (India) Pvt Ltd
Muskaan Complex, Plot No. 3, B-2, Vasant Kunj, New Delhi – 110070, India

Hay House LLC, P.O. Box 5100, Carlsbad, CA 92018-5100, USA
Hay House UK Ltd, 1st Floor, Crawford Corner, 91-93 Baker Street, London W1U 6QQ, UK
Hay House Australia Publishing Pty Ltd, 18/36 Ralph St., Alexandria NSW 2015, Australia

Email: contact@hayhouse.co.in
Website: www.hayhouse.co.in

First published by Hay House India, 2025
10 9 8 7 6 5 4 3 2 1

ISBN 978-93-6611-131-5
ISBN 978-93-6611-791-1 (E-Book)

Printed at Replika Press Pvt Ltd

FSC www.fsc.org MIX Paper | Supporting responsible forestry FSC™ C016779

Hay House is committed to a sustainable future for our business, our readers and our planet. This book is made from Forest Stewardship Council® certified paper.

A well-researched book on the physiological and biochemical functioning and impact of yogic asanas. This will serve as an excellent reference book for yoga instructors as well as curious yoga asana practitioners. The last section on FAQ and myths about Yoga practice is nicely put together and helpful.

—Ami Ganatra,
Author of *Mahabharata Unravelled* & *Ramayana Unravelled*

As a yoga researcher, I commend *The Yoga Science* for its invaluable achievement in offering yoga practitioners much-needed clarity on asanas, debunking myths, exploring yogic applications, and much more. From any dimension you approach yogic ecology, this comprehensive guide has it all.

—Satyam Tiwari
Scientist and Senior Research Fellow, IIT Mandi

Divyansh Sharma's rigorous analysis of yoga, combining ancient wisdom with a contemporary scientific approach, exemplifies the problem-solving methods used by leading researchers. By bridging the gap between traditional practice and modern scientific inquiry, Sharma illuminates the potential for innovation that emerges when diverse disciplines intersect. This book will be a significant addition to the body of knowledge.

—Dr Gourav Dwivedi
Assistant Professor, IIT Delhi

Whether you're a beginner or an advanced practitioner, *The Yoga Science* offers something for everyone. Highly recommended for those looking not just to practise yoga, but to embrace it as a way of life.

—Dr Vidhey Tirpude
Assistant Professor, Department of Surgery,
Government Medical College, Gondia, Maharashtra

To
Adiyogi, the first yogi,
the Himalayas, bearer of timeless wisdom,
and my Nana ji.

Contents

Section III
Untwining the Asanas

Section IV
The Final Stretch

Foreword

Hearty congratulations on this impressive work and outstanding contribution to the world of Yoga! This book is a shining example of reverence for ancient traditions seamlessly blended with contemporary scientific insights. Divyansh's unique approach masterfully integrates yoga with biomechanics and research, offering practical solutions for beginners, in-depth insights for seasoned practitioners, and comprehensive guidance for holistic health and well-being.

The research-backed benefits of yoga on every organ and system are meticulously presented. I particularly appreciate the thoughtful sections addressing FAQs and debunking myths, which adeptly tackle common challenges faced by practitioners. The detailed descriptions of each asana, accompanied by line diagrams, potential benefits, modifications, and biomechanics, make this guide an invaluable resource for practitioners of all levels.

This comprehensive guide provides practical solutions for those seeking to explore unique dimensions of yoga. I highly recommend this book to anyone looking to deepen their understanding of yoga's transformative power through a scientific lens.

Best wishes,

—Dr Ishwar V. Basavaraddi
Former Director, Morarji National Institute of Yoga,
Ministry of Ayush, Government of India, New Delhi
18 November 2024

Preface

Why Yoga?

When searching for the best-suited exercise regime, factors like calorie expenditure, functionality, injury prevention, stronger muscles, personalisation based on bio-individuality, fluidity, and stress reduction are instrumental. Yoga excels in all these factors with flying colours. This book will thoroughly dive deeper and help you understand the role of yoga with relevant research. Yoga, especially vinyasa and sun salutations, can burn more than 400 calories per hour, higher than basketball, tennis, callisthenics, and strength training (Gordon 2014; Joshua and Dunbar 2016; Carroll et al. 2003). In terms of functionality, yoga mimics real-life body movements and is safer than machine-based exercises, primarily because the sense of joint positioning (proprioception) supersedes and prevents injuries, whereas machine-based exercises have more risk of injuries (Maior and de Assis 2023). For those who strictly need aesthetic gains and enhanced muscle mass, I recommend a 'muscular yoga' regime where dumbbells, barbells, resistance bands, etc. can be integrated. However, it goes against the conventional approach. Based on needs, exercises should be personalised—with more modifications, yoga can accommodate more individuals and perform better than other physical exercises (Govindaraj et al. 2016, 242–53). Beyond physical realms, yoga's mental, social, and spiritual gains are unparalleled. As you will witness throughout the book, yoga is an ancient wisdom relevant to date with the backing of science and many proven benefits.

The Idea of this Book: After going through an 15-year-long yogic journey and learning yoga from reputed teachers and institutions, I found several contradictions in perceived yoga alignment, science, and more. The differences became stark based on institution, style, and place. I found my fellow yogis to be travelling in the same boat. This paved the way for my personal research, which took four more years. This book is an attempt to demystify and visualise the understanding of yoga concerning biomechanics, anatomy, and physiology that I learnt through consistent endeavours, gurus, reading several research journals, ancient yogic texts, contemporary science books, and more.

My Personal Journey: A sports injury—right after discovering yoga—could not prevent me from embracing it. Persistent, I developed my yoga practice to the point I could perform Urdhva Mukha Vrksasana (Handstand Pose), an advanced balancing asana. For the next few years, I bonded well with most asanas. Yet, life intervened, I was pulled to the paths of science and engineering, and my journey of yoga was temporarily halted. In my engineering years, when life struck me with multiple challenges and depression, I rekindled my love for yoga. It changed my world to be more vibrant and livelier than ever before.

What to Expect: Through this book, we will embark on a journey into the world of yoga, bridging ancient science with contemporary science and uncovering its underlying mechanisms. While a multitude of research has shown yoga to be effective across most health parameters, much of its potential is clouded due to the widespread mysticism backed by unsupported claims. This book unearths the anatomy, physiology, and biomechanics of yoga while retaining its rich legacy. Furthermore, we will learn about more than 50 asanas, well-suited for beginners and advanced practitioners alike. Whether you are an enthusiast or professional this comprehensive book will guide you to elevate your knowledge and practice of yoga, backed by research and ancient scriptures.

Namaste!

Introduction

Awakening the Yogic Way

Have you wondered how yoga, a 5,000-year-old ancient science, can empower you with its undeniable benefits? Imagine a more resilient, active, healthy, and serene life. However, how can yoga unlock the hidden potential within you? How did ancient yogis design yoga? With this segment, let's commence the yogic journey while navigating through the various yogic scriptures and understanding yoga's ancient roots.

Meaning of Yoga

Yuj Samyoge

'Yoga' is derived from the Sanskrit root word *Yuj*—which means 'to join' or 'to yoke' or 'to unite'. The union of a being with the Supreme Being is called 'yoga'. Primarily, this definition arises from Vyasa Bhasya. However, apart from this definition, we also have a few other definitions that interpret yoga differently. In this segment, we will discuss more traditional definitions of yoga directly from various yogic scriptures:

a. Discipline in action is yoga

   Atha Yogānuśāsanam [1.1]

   According to the Patanjali yoga Sutras, the correct meaning of this shloka is 'now, we will start the discipline of yoga'. However, people often interpret it as 'the discipline in our actions is yoga'.

b. Cessation of fluctuations of the mind is yoga (Patanjali Yoga Sutra)

Yogaśchittavṛttinirodhaḥ [1.2]

Yoga is the cessation of the ripples of the *Chitta* (intellect or mind).

c. Liberation is yoga (Vyasa Bhasya)

Yogah Samadhi

Liberation from our karmic imprints is yoga. Here, karmic imprints mean actions that lead to good or bad results.

d. Detachment from results and equanimity is yoga (Shrimad Bhagavad Gita)

Yogastha: Kuru Karmani Sangam Tyktva Dhananjay.
Siddhyasiddhyo: Samo Bhootva Samatvam Yoga Uchyate [2.48]

O Arjuna, abandon impurities, attachment of success, failure, or otherwise. The Equanimity of mind free from desires and expectations is yoga.

e. Skill in action is yoga (Shrimad Bhagavad Gita)

Buddhi Yukto Jahatiha Ubhe Sukrita-Dushkrite
Tasmad Yogaya Yujyasva Yogah Karmasu Kaushalam [2.50]

The man who fulfils his obligation with Nishkama karma (desireless actions) goes beyond good and bad. Thus, seek Nishkama karma with an equanimous mind. Yoga is skill in action.

Basics of Yoga

When you are a beginner, you are filled with endless questions—where to practise, when to eat, when to drink water, which mat to buy, and a lot more. In this segment, we will try to answer relevant questions from a beginner's standpoint.

What to Wear

While practising yoga, opt for breathable, loose, and comfortable clothes that allow for freedom of movement and enable the body to release heat and sweat efficiently. Selecting such attire ensures that your focus remains on your practice without distractions, as restrictive clothing can impede the flow of energy and limit your range of motion.

Which Yoga Mat to Use

The first step is to buy a good quality yoga mat. Typically, a standard yoga mat is about 2 feet in width and 6 feet in length. However, larger options are also available. Several factors should be considered while purchasing a yoga mat—quality, durability, comfort, material, and grip (anti-skid). Let's briefly look at some of the vital factors:

a. **Material Matters**

   Typically, TPE (Thermoplastic Elastomer), natural rubber, or PVC-free materials are considered viable options. They are mostly recyclable and/or environmentally friendly.

b. **Thickness of the Mat**

   The thickness of the yoga mat is also an essential aspect to look for. While deciding the thickness you may ask yourself whether to choose comfort or portability. I suggest choosing the former. Comfort should be the criterion for a safe yoga practice. However, for hygiene issues, people often go for thin mats to pair with the mats provided by yoga studios.

c. **Grip Strength**

The Grip of the mat is another important factor. A good grip helps to stabilise and prevent injuries. Anti-skid mats are best suited in this regard. Ensure your mat has a grip on both sides. Lastly, your mat should provide a good grip even when you are sweating.

Where to Practise

You can practise yoga in a well-ventilated space. Various Hatha yogic scriptures suggest choosing a place that is neither too windy nor completely still. Furthermore, the environment should be clean and free from pollution. The area should be well-lit and away from distractions. The greener the better as the colour green is soothing for the eyes. Following the traditional yogic approach, the aim is to turn inward, so it is recommended to avoid mirrors.

When to Practise

According to most yogic scriptures, the Brahmamuhurta (pre-dawn) is seen as the best time to practise yoga. However, based on the current lifestyle we lead, it may not be feasible for many of us. In such cases, you can practise either in the morning or evening.

When to Eat

Before practising a physical form of yoga, keep your stomach empty for 3–4 hours after a heavy meal and 1–2 hours after a light meal.

When to Drink Water

You can drink water whenever you want during the yoga session. In fact, it is essential for us to remain hydrated during a yoga class. Proper hydration helps in:

- Decreasing core temperature
- Optimal muscle functioning
- Preventing exhaustion
- Eliminating toxins
- Balancing fluids
- Preventing cramps and injuries

When to Bathe

The second limb of Patanjali's Ashtanga yoga (eight limb yoga) starts with *shaucha*, which means cleanliness. Therefore, you should ideally clean yourself and eliminate waste from your body before attempting yoga.

The Need for Foundation

I remember attending a product innovation meeting for the yoga category of one of the world's largest sports brands. Everyone present was a seasoned yoga professional. Despite this, many were clueless about the quality and material of the yoga products being discussed. This intrigued me, and I thought about how difficult it would be for beginners and enthusiasts to select the right attire, yoga mat, and other essentials. In this chapter we covered the foundational aspects of yoga, so you do not need to learn it the hard way. Whether you are starting or deep into the practice, these insights will guide you to focus on your goal.

Section I
The Ancient Science of Yoga

Yoga has a history of over 5000 years. The credit for yoga's survival must be given to the Ancient Science of yoga. While some concepts of yoga have been demystified, there is still so much more to unearth. In this segment, we will discuss the ancient science of yoga from its original sources along with Shlokas, Mantras, and Sutras.

1

From Ancient Texts to Modern Practice: The Evolution of Yoga

3300 BCE: Indus Saraswati Valley Civilisation

The history of yoga goes back well beyond 5,000–8,000 years. Archaeologists have recovered numerous seals and fossils from the Indus Saraswati Valley Civilisation (3300–1300 BCE) that depict yogic practices. There are two primary stories surrounding the originator of yoga. According to one story, Hiranyagarbha was the originator of yoga. If we break down the word Hiranyagarbha, we get *Hiranya*, which means 'golden', and *Garbha*, which means 'womb'. The golden womb is believed to be the creator of the entire universe. The story of Hiranyagarbha is strikingly similar to the concept of the Big Bang Theory. According to another story, Lord Shiva, or Adiyogi, is the originator of yoga. Irrespective of the version, yogic practices are considered more spiritual than religious.

1800 BCE: Rig Veda

The first known mention of the term 'yoga' is found in the Rig Veda. The Rig Veda is one of the oldest pieces of literature ever discovered. However, the Agama system was prevalent in the Indus Saraswati Valley civilisation. Agama was a tradition wherein one generation would transfer all their knowledge to the next generation through oral communication. Therefore, determining the exact time period of the Rig Veda is almost impossible.

500 BCE: Shrimad Bhagavad Gita

The Shrimad Bhagavad Gita is believed to have come into existence around 500 BCE. It is based on the conversation between Lord Krishna and Arjuna. Interestingly, all the chapters end with the term 'yoga'. Moreover, the entire scripture avidly describes yoga, primarily discussing jnana yoga (knowledge yoga), karma yoga (action yoga), samkhya yoga (analytical yoga), abhyasa yoga (practice yoga), and bhakti yoga (devotional yoga).

500–200 BCE: Maharshi Patanjali's Yoga Darshan

The practice of yoga continued to flourish over thousands of years. According to some estimates, Maharshi Patanjali's Yoga Darshan emerged around 200 BCE. Yoga Darshan explores yoga through various *sutras* (codifications or formulations). Although online sources often suggest Maharshi Patanjali was the originator of yoga, he was not. He clarifies this in the very first sutra. The Patanjali Yoga Sutra, often referred to as the Yoga Sutra of Patanjali, is considered the most authentic text on yoga.

9th Century CE: Goraksha Shataka and Siddha Siddhanta Paddhati

In the 9th century CE, Guru Goraksha Natha is said to have written the Goraksha Samhita, which is the first known written evidence of hatha yoga. Guru Goraksha Natha was a disciple of Guru Matsyendra Natha. Hatha yoga revolutionised the world of yoga forever. The contemporary physical form of yoga is mostly based on hatha yoga. Guru Goraksha Natha also wrote several other important texts on yoga, including Goraksha Shataka and Siddha Siddhanta Paddhati.

13th Century CE: Shiva Samhita

In the 13th century CE, another ancient yogic scripture, Shiva Samhita (Shiva's Compendium), is thought to have come into existence. This text introduced four asanas. It is based on the conversations between Lord Shiva and his consort, Parvati. It also discusses mudras, the importance of a guru, *siddhi*, and visualisation. However, the author of this text remains unknown.

15th Century CE: Hatha Yoga Pradipika

In the 15th century CE, another key ancient yogic scripture came into existence, known as Hatha Pradipika or Hatha Yoga Pradipika (light on hatha yoga). This text was written by Swami Svatmarama, a disciple of Guru Goraksha Natha's tradition. The Hatha Yoga Pradipika describes four limbs of yoga: Asana, pranayama, mudra (gesture), and Nadaanusandhana (meditation). It outlines 15 asanas in total.

17th Century CE: Gheranda Samhita

In the 17th century CE, two invaluable hatha yogic scriptures emerged—the Gheranda Samhita and the Hatha Ratnavali. The Gheranda Samhita (Gheranda's Compendium) was written by Maharshi Gheranda. It discusses the seven limbs of yoga, namely shatkarma (cleansing), Asana (yoga posture), mudra (gestures), pratyahara (withdrawal of senses), pranayama (breathing techniques), dhyana (meditation), and samadhi (liberation). The gheranda samhita describes 32 asanas.

On the other hand, the Hatha Ratnavali was written by Srinivasa, which describes 84 asanas. It is noteworthy that while most hatha yogic scriptures refer to 84 Asanas, only the Hatha Ratnavali lists all of them.

ASANA: THE ORIGINS

Earliest Records of the History of Asana

The importance of asanas is evident in most yogic traditions. Evidence of asanas being used as part of the yogic regime can be traced to ancient Indian civilisation. In some ancient depictions, dated to around 3300 BCE, yogic postures were carved. The special Pashupati seal of the Indus-Saraswati Valley Civilisation shows Pashupati assuming Mulabandhasana (Root Lock Pose).

Patanjali's Yoga Sutra

Patanjali's Yoga Sutra (c. 500–200 BCE) mentions asana in 2.46. However, according to many yoga scholars, Maharshi Patanjali is only referring to the dhyanatmak asanas (meditative postures).

The Inception of Hatha Yoga

Despite the depiction of asanas, whether the people of the Indus-Saraswati Valley Civilisation practised more physically advanced asanas is debatable. It is believed that more physically advanced asanas were introduced with the inception of hatha yoga. Various hatha yogic scriptures mention asanas that are still practised today.

Goraksha Sataka and Siddha Siddhanta Paddhati

In the 9th century CE, Guru Goraksha Natha wrote Goraksha Sataka, Goraksha Samhita, Siddha Siddhanta Paddhati, Yoga Siddhanta Paddhati, etc. Guru Goraksha Natha describes six limbs of yoga in the Goraksha Sataka as follows:

> *Asanam pranasyamah pratyaharotha dharana.*
> *Dhyanam samadhiretani yogagani bhavanti shat* [7]

He describes these limbs as: Asana (posture), pranasamrodha (breath restraint), pratyahara (withdrawal of senses), dharana (concentration), dhyana (meditation or absorption), and samadhi (enlightenment or liberation). He equates the number of asanas to the number of species present.

Shiva Samhita

The Shiva Samhita was written around the 13th century CE. The text discusses various limbs of yoga, such as asana, mudra, chakras, and mantras. The Shiva Samhita refers to 84 major asanas, of which it mentions only four, as described in the following shloka:

Chaturshityasanani santi nanavidhani cha
Tebhya schatushkamadaya mayoktani bravimayam.
Siddhasanam tah padmasanan chogran cha swastikam [3.100]

It identifies the four most important asanas: Siddhasana (Accomplished Pose), Padmasana (Lotus Pose), Ugrasana (Paschimottanasana or Seated Forward Bend Pose), and Swastikasana (Auspicious Pose).

Hatha Yoga Pradipika

The Hatha Yoga Pradipika is estimated to have been written in the 15th century CE by Swami Svatmarama. It describes four limbs of yoga—the first chapter covers the principles of yoga and asanas, the second chapter focuses on satkarma (cleansing practices) and pranayama (breathing techniques), the third chapter discusses mudras (gestures, locks, or seals), and the fourth chapter details samadhi (enlightenment or liberation). The Hatha Yoga Pradipika mentions 15 asanas, many of which are covered in the text.

Gheranda Samhita

The Gheranda Samhita is believed to have originated around the 17th century CE, written by Maharshi Gheranda. It describes the seven limbs of yoga—shatkarma (cleansing practices), asana (yoga posture), mudra (gestures, locks, or seals), pratyahara (withdrawal of senses), pranayama (breath techniques), dhyana (meditation or absorption), and samadhi (liberation or enlightenment). The Gheranda Samhita mentions 32 asanas in total, some of which have already been covered in this book.

HATHA YOGA STYLES

The physical form of hatha yoga is often practised in various styles, which have gained traction for a few decades. Here, we will briefly discuss these styles and the calories they burn.

One thing is certain, some yoga forms burn more calories than typical cardio or aerobic exercises. Therefore, if your goal is to lose excess fat, you can choose any yogic form according to your body type and suitability. Please do not only go for calorie intake while opting for a yoga class; instead, look beyond aesthetics and calorie burn. Choose a style that has a holistic approach. Keep your overall health in mind.

Traditional Hatha Yoga

Hatha yoga is a traditional form of yoga, all asanas falling under it. In traditional hatha yoga, the postures are typically held for 10 seconds to 5 minutes.

Burns 180–250 calories per hour session.

Vinyasa Yoga (Flow Yoga)

Vinyasa yoga is also called 'flow yoga'. Here, we flow from one pose into the other with the synchronisation of breath. It was started by Tirumalai Krishnamacharya. He was the guru of K. Pattabhi Jois and was related to B. K. S. Iyengar. Here, asanas are held for not more than five seconds or breaths.

Burns 400–600 calories per hour session.

Ashtanga Vinyasa (Masoor Style Yoga or Power Yoga)

Ashtanga Vinyasa is a practice of hatha yoga, which was popularised by K. Pattabhi Jois. He named it Ashtanga yoga because he fused Ashtanga yoga (eight limbs of Yoga) and vinyasa yoga.

Burns 420–580 calories per hour session.

Hot Yoga

Hot yoga is more popular in the western hemisphere where the temperature is comparatively lower. Here, the yoga studio is kept at 39–42 degrees Celsius.

Burns 350–450 calories per hour session.

Yin Yoga

Yin yoga was popularised by Taoist yoga teacher Paulie Zink. It is also a style based on hatha yoga. Here, postures are held for a longer period, about 3–5 minutes.

Restorative Yoga

Restorative yoga is based on the teaching of B. K. S. Iyengar. Here, the idea is to relax our entire body without stretching too much. Here, postures are held for an extended period, about 5–10 minutes.

THE RICH TAPESTRY OF YOGA PRACTICES

Pranayama

Prana means vital energy or life force; *Ayama* translates to regulation or dimension.

The translation of pranayama is the regulation of prana with the help of breath. Pranayama is often also depicted as kumbhaka or kumbhaka yoga. Pranayama is an integral limb of yoga, and its practice is believed to be as old as asanas. Early depictions of pranayama can be found in the Shrimad Bhagavad Gita and Patanjali's Yoga Sutra. Both of these ancient texts are estimated to have been written around 500–200 BCE.

Mudras

Mudra is translated as gesture, seal, or lock. Mudras have always been a part of hatha yogic practices. One of the definitions found in the prominent scripture Shiv Samhita is as follows:

Ishvara Uvaach
Athaatah Sampravakshyami Mudrikayogamuttamam
Tasya Abhyaasamatren Sarvavyaadhih Pramuchyate [4.1]

In this *shloka*, it is stated that practising *mudras* can potentially free us from various diseases.

If we notice, gestures have always been an integral part of our lives. Every tradition embraces gestures in one way or another. Ancient yogis seem to have been aware of the connection between our brains and the gestures we perform. This is possibly why they experimented with gestures to channel our dormant energies.

Mudras, though more ancient, supposedly work on principles similar to acupressure. However, according to yogic philosophy, mudras help to channel or redirect the flow of prana. Mudras are divided into several categories, such as hasta mudra (hand gesture), kaya mudra (bodily mudras), bandha mudra (locks), mana mudras (mudras for the mind), and adhara mudra (pelvic mudras).

Mantra

One of the definitions of mantra is: *Mananāt Trāyatē Iti Mantrah*

The simplest definition of *mantra* is 'may it protect'. A mantra is defined as 'a chant, the utterance or contemplation of which releases one from the eternal cycle of birth and death'.

The practice of mantra or mantra yoga is primarily designed for people who believe in a supreme being. In Vedic tradition, mantras are considered to be a part of the Vedas. It is believed that every mantra contains an invaluable power to grant what we desire. In one way or another, mantras later became popular in various other traditions as well.

According to scholars, mantras hold a science of their own. The concept of mantra is possibly based on one of two principles. First, the dual nature of particles, i.e., both particle and wave nature. Second, the principle of vibration, which states that everything is moving and has certain vibrations. When we practise mantra yoga, we try to signal the universe to fill us with subtle energies that grant our wishes.

To practise mantra yoga, you can assume any dhyanatmak asana (meditative pose). You can also use the mudra of your choice. It is believed that each mantra generates a specific vibration. Some of these vibrations supposedly match the vibrations of certain cosmic activities. However, more rigorous research is needed to support these claims. Furthermore, according to some prominent yogis, it is important to practise mantra yoga under the guidance of a qualified yoga teacher.

Dharana (Concentration, Visualisation, and Mindfulness)

Dharana is an umbrella term that covers three aspects: Concentration, visualisation, and mindfulness. One aspect, mindfulness, is about being in the present, noticing the fluctuations of the mind, body, and surroundings without judgement. Mindfulness is becoming more popular by the day. Plenty of evidence suggests that mindfulness is a proven technique for reducing anxiety and stress. A study recently concluded that mindfulness-based stress reduction is as effective as the antidepressant escitalopram (Hoge et al., 2023).

Dhyana (Meditation)

Meditation has also gained traction in recent years because of its numerous benefits. There are different types of meditation, but primarily there are two: Open monitoring (OM) meditation and focused attention (FA) meditation. In open monitoring meditation, the meditator observes their surroundings or things that are subject to change, while in focused attention meditation, awareness is locked onto a single object of meditation.

Contemporary medicine is gradually recognising the importance of meditation. It is linked to many evidence-based benefits, including its ability to rewire our brain, a process known as neuroplasticity (Tolahunase, 2018; Guidotti et al., 2021). Moreover, meditation offers solutions to many problems associated with our modern lifestyle.

2

Ashtanga Yoga: Embracing Eight Limbs of Progression

Ashtanga yoga is translated as the eight limbs of yoga (*Ashta* = Eight, *Anga* = Limbs). Please do not confuse it with Ashtanga Vinyasa, which borrows Ashtanga yoga from Maharshi Patanjali's Yoga Darshan. Maharshi Patanjali is believed to have existed between 500 and 200 BCE. As we know, Maharshi Patanjali wrote the Yoga Darshan, where he mentions various forms of yoga. One of the forms that Maharshi Patanjali recommends for beginners is Ashtanga yoga.

> *Yama-Niyama-Asana-Pranayama-Pratyahara-Dharana-Dhyana-Samadhi Ashtav-Angani* [2.29]

Through this shloka, Maharshi describes Ashtanga yoga as follows: Yama, niyama, asana, pranayama, pratyahara, dharana, dhyana, and samadhi. According to many scholars, Ashtanga yoga is depicted chronologically.

Moral Ethics: Yama

Yama, the first limb, represents moral ethics. These are moral codes that one should follow. I believe yama includes principles that one should observe for a better society. Maharshi Patanjali describes yama through the following shloka:

> *Ahimsa-Satya-Asteya-Brahmacharya-Aparigrahah Yamah* [2.30]

Here, he says yama can be further divided into five moral codes, which are as follows (yama should be followed in three ways—mentally, verbally, and physically):

- *Ahimsa* = Non-violence
- *Satya* = Truthfulness
- *Asteya* = Non-stealing
- *Brahmacharya* = Celibacy, balance
- *Aparigraha* = Non-possessiveness

Self-Observance: Niyama

Niyama, the second limb, represents self-observance. These are self-disciplinary actions that benefit our learning abilities and lead to spiritual ethics. Maharshi Patanjali describes Niyama through the following shloka:

Shaucha-Santosha-Tapah-Svadhyaya-Ishvarapranidhanani Niyamah [2.32]

Here, he says niyama can be further divided into five self-observances:

- *Shaucha* = Cleanliness
- *Santosha* = Contentment
- *Tapah* = Austerity
- *Swadhyaya* = Self-study
- *Ishvara Pranidhana* = Surrender to the Supreme

Yoga Posture: Asana

Asana is the third limb of Patanjali's Ashtanga yoga. Asana is indeed an invaluable aspect of yoga. In the contemporary context, when we think of asanas, we think of bodily postures.

However, it is important to note that the Asanas Maharshi Patanjali mentions in the Yoga Darshan do not include all physical postures; he was likely referring to meditative postures. Maharshi Patanjali describes asana through the following shloka:

Sthira-Sukham Asanam [2.46]

Here, he says asana is any stance or posture in which you experience joy and stability.

Regulation of Breath: Pranayama

Pranayama is the fourth limb of Patanjali's Ashtanga yoga. As we know, pranayama refers to breathing techniques that regulate the breath in a healthy manner. Maharshi Patanjali describes pranayama through the following shloka:

Tasmin Sati Shvasa-Prashvasayoh Gativicchedah Pranayamah [2.49]

Here, he says, when you control your inhalation or exhalation from its usual course, it is pranayama. In the following shlokas, Maharshi Patanjali mentions four types of pranayama: Bahya vritti, abhyantara vritti, stambha vritti, and chaturtha:

Bahya Abhyantara Stambha Vrttir Desha Kala Samkhyabhih Paridrsto Dirghasuksmah [2.50]

[The regulation of breath, both external and internal, and the suspension of breath should be observed with regard to place, time, and number, becoming prolonged and subtle.]

Bahya-Abhyantara-Visayakshepi Chaturthah [2.51]

[The fourth type (of breath regulation) transcends external and internal objects.]

Sense Withdrawal: Pratyahara

Pratyahara is the fifth limb of Patanjali's Ashtanga yoga. Pratyahara is a way to withdraw our senses. As we know, our sensory organs constantly seek external stimulation. According to yogic philosophy, such stimulation ultimately leads to sorrow. Maharshi Patanjali describes pratyahara through the following shloka:

Sva-Vishaya-Samprayoge Citta-Svarupanukara
Ivendriyanam Pratyahara [2.54]

Here, he says that when our sensory organs are withdrawn from external stimuli and guided by the mind, it is Pratyahara.

Mindfulness or Concentration: Dharana

Dharana is the sixth limb of Patanjali's Ashtanga yoga. It is also known as mindfulness or concentration. In dharana, we keep our minds focused on something for a short period. Maharshi Patanjali describes dharana through the following shloka:

Desha-Bandhas Chittasya Dharana [3.1]

Here, he says focusing your mind on a particular point for a short time is dharana.

Meditation: Dhyana

Dhyana is the seventh limb of Patanjali's Ashtanga yoga. Dhyana is also known as absorption or meditation. Unlike dharana, dhyana lasts longer, and the practitioner becomes absorbed in the object of meditation. Maharshi Patanjali describes dhyana through the following shloka:

Tatra Pratyaya-Ekatanata Dhyana [3.2]

Through this shloka, Maharshi says that when we remain

in a state of focused attention for an extended time, it becomes dhyana.

Liberation or Enlightenment: Samadhi

Samadhi is the eighth and final limb of Patanjali's Ashtanga yoga. It can be translated as liberation or enlightenment. Samadhi is the ultimate stage of yoga, where one detaches from the eternal cycle of life and death. This is considered the highest state of realisation. Maharshi Patanjali describes samadhi through the following shloka:

> *Tadevartha-Matra-Nirbhāsam Svarupa-Shunyamiva Samadhih* [3.3]
>
> Maharshi says that when only the object of meditation remains and everything else, including the self, disappears, that state is samadhi.

Section II

Anatomy, Physiology, and Biomechanics of Yoga

Doctors are prescribing yoga more than ever. Do you wonder why? What is the exact science behind yoga? Anatomy is the branch of science that focuses on human structure, whereas physiology focuses on various body components that interact with each other. In this segment, we will examine several studies to draw parallels between the anatomy, physiology, and biomechanics of yoga while deriving information through research articles. We will also learn how yoga science is not limited to the physical realms but also the mental, social, and transcendental ones.

3
The Science-Backed Power of Yoga

Yoga offers profound benefits, of which we have only scratched the surface. Those who have practised yoga even once can vouch for its remarkable healing and energising qualities. It changed how I used to perceive things, but now I empathise with those who still require evidence before trusting anything. This is precisely why I wrote this book. Throughout this book, we will observe the benefits of various Yogic practices. Curious minds cannot be satisfied without proper explanations of benefits; therefore, I am presenting some of the widespread benefits of yoga along with their mechanisms.

Strengthens Muscles

People believe yoga is all about mere stretching, however, there is more to it than what meets the eye. Yoga releases and strengthens our tightened muscles (Lau, Yu, and Woo 2015). Yoga is a body-mass exercise where our muscles contract in all possible ways to sustain various yoga postures against gravity. Furthermore, yoga practices can also be modified to strengthen more muscles.

Enhances Flexibility

Most people opt to practise yoga for enhanced flexibility. A study concluded that yoga was quite effective in improving our overall flexibility (Petric, Vauhnik, and Jakovljevic

2014). Hatha yoga can also increase the flexibility of our legs, thighs, hip flexors, and chest muscles. The same study also concluded Hatha yoga's significance in enhancing joint health.

Calms the Mind

Most yoga practices activate the parasympathetic nervous system (PNS) response and downregulate the sympathetic nervous system (SNS) response of the body. The PNS is a part of the nervous system that calms the body and mind. When we practise yoga, it regulates the body's stress response (SNS) (Chin and Kales 2019).

Improves Digestion

Yoga can also be effective in easing our digestive system. The reason, again, is the PNS activation, which controls the rest and digest response. A study (Ganesh, Subramanya, and Udupa 2021) also concluded yoga is effective in improving digestion in senior citizens.

Enhances Respiratory Health

A study (Chanavirut et al., 2006) has presented that yoga can expand our chest walls. Therefore, it gives more space for the lungs to expand, contributing to improved respiratory system. It is likely due to the increased strength of our respiratory muscles that lift our skeletal structure to give more room to the respiratory organs.

Increases Mobility and Functional Fitness

Yoga can improve joint mobility by mobilising various connective tissues surrounding our synovial joints (movable joints). Furthermore, with the mobilisation of our joints, practising yoga can significantly improve our functional fitness

(Gothe and McAuley 2016). This means our motion becomes more efficient with yoga.

Supports Fat Loss

Yoga supports fat loss by moving the larger muscles of the body. When we practise yoga, the body needs more energy, which is ultimately fulfilled by our stored energy (fat or carbohydrates). To utilise this stored energy, our body increases Oxygen demand. Thus, yoga also helps shred fat by forcing our body into aerobic (with oxygen) respiration. (Ross et al., 2016).

Reduces Stress, Anxiety, and Depression

Our lives are becoming incrementally more stressful and sedentary. Our body greatly depends on physical activities to cope with stress. However, these days, we barely move, which substantially diminishes our ability to cope with stress, anxiety, and depression. Yoga can help prevent and/or overcome such psychosomatic disorders (Singphow et al., 2022) by working on our nervous and endocrine systems.

Boosts Immunity

In a systematic review, it was concluded that yoga helps to reduce the activity of pro-inflammatory markers (Falkenberg, Eising, Peters 2018). As we know, inflammation can weaken our immune system. Furthermore, yoga reduces stress and improves perceived quality of life, sleep quality, and beyond—all of which are known to contribute to better immunity.

Increases Bone Mineral Density

As we age, we lose bone mineral density due to various factors. Loss of bone mineral density is more prevalent in postmenopausal women, and practising yoga can improve one's bone mineral density (Lu et al., 2015) as it is an isometric resistance exercise (Hong and Kim 2018).

Promotes Better Equilibrioception (Balance) and Proprioception (Body Awareness)

Yoga involves assuming various balance-centric asanas and practices. These practices are often linked with an improved sense of equilibrioception and proprioception. A study on visually impaired students concluded that yoga is indeed helpful in improving proprioception (Mohanty, Pradhan, and Nagathna 2014). This means we can prevent hurting our little toes with better body awareness.

Protects the Joints

Yoga can be instrumental in protecting our joints by engaging our muscles. Various yogic practices are less intense and can also strengthen specific muscle groups in isolation, giving yoga an additional advantage over other forms of exercise in joint protection and rehabilitation. Muscle strengthening works in several ways, including joint and spine stabilisation, shock absorption, improved range of motion, better muscle firing rate, and enhanced proprioception. All these factors are present in Yoga, making it an appealing option for joint injury prevention and rehabilitation. However, for optimal results, it can also be combined with physiotherapy.

Restores Homeostasis

Homeostasis is the body's ability to keep the body healthy while maintaining a normalised and balanced state. It was concluded in a study that Yoga can maintain immune homeostasis in people with rheumatoid arthritis (Gautam et al. 2023).

Improves Overall Posture

Yoga can improve our overall posture by strengthening the muscles that surround our spine, shoulders, and hip joints. When we strengthen these muscles, they stabilise the joints, in turn, improving one's overall posture.

Helps Manage High Blood Pressure

Yoga can also help to manage blood pressure, especially in someone with hypertension. A systematic review concluded that yoga significantly helps lower blood pressure in hypertensive and prehypertensive individuals as compared to no treatment at all (Hagins, Selfe, and Innes 2013).

4

The Many Dimensions of Health

Our health is the most valuable thing to us, above all else. Yet, many of us take it for granted. There are numerous aspects of health that we need to monitor. To achieve this, we need to recognise that our body is the only means through which we interact with the outside world. If we neglect our bodies, we won't be able to live happily or fulfil our responsibilities. This idea is also expressed by the Sanskrit intellectual, Shri Kalidasa, who writes in Sarga 5:33 of Kumarasambhavam.

शरीरमाद्यं खलु धर्मसाधनम् [5:33]

Shariramadyam Khalu Dharmasadhanam [5:33]

It means, our body is an invaluable medium through which we fulfil our (good) deeds.

It is widely believed that our overall health is a reflection of various aspects of it. According to the World Health Organisation (WHO, 1946), there are three dimensions of overall health: Physical, mental, and social; not the mere absence of disease. However, according to practitioners from the yogic ecosystem and spiritual health, other yogic health parameters are equally vital. Therefore, in this section, we will discuss the dimensions of overall health:

- Physical health (WHO)
- Mental health (WHO)

- Social health (WHO)
- Spiritual health (yogic ecosystem)
- Yogic transcendental health (yogic ecosystem)

It is worth noting that these dimensions of health are interlinked. Thus, instability in one dimension can have a cascading effect.

Physical Health

When an individual is free from physical diseases (*vyadhi*) and can do his/her regular deeds without any ailment, fatigue, injury, etc., then they are physically healthy. Furthermore, physical health is often also looked at from the kinesiology perspective where the motion, forces, and mechanics concerning the human body is observed, combined with anatomy, physiology, and psychology. Therefore, assessing our body through kinesiology can help us understand overall physical health.

Physiological Health

Physiological health is concerned with how our body processes certain operations. For instance, we could be physically healthy, but our digestion could be disrupted. Similarly, other physiological disorders can also hinder our health related to any our organ system. Harmony between these systems ensures proper physiological and physical health. Physiological health is a subset of physical health.

Mental Health

Mental health is more about our minds, thoughts, emotions, and feelings. It is the combination of cognitive abilities, psychological health, behavioural health, and emotional health.

Cognitive health includes thinking, reasoning, problem-solving, and decision-making. Moreover, mental health is greatly intertwined with physical health more than we think it is. WHO insinuates mental well-being as a state without any mental disease along with the ability to counter stress, build relationships, cater to your community, learn, and work well.

Psychological Health

Psychological health is a reflection of emotional, mental, social, and spiritual health. It is usually considered a subset of mental health.

Emotional Health

Emotional health is linked with how we perceive things around us. It is also dependent on how likely we associate and cope with positive and negative emotions. Emotional health is also usually considered a part of mental health.

Social Health

Social health is invaluable to humans. People seldom realise that we have developed such advanced brains because we learnt the power of communication, community defence, competition, and interdependence (Connor 2007, 587–602). Therefore, in a way, it can be concluded that human intelligence greatly depends on socialisation and communication. This also insinuates that our health depends on forging relationships, building communication, interacting with others, and more. I believe this is also why we inherited behavioural patterns of helping others, even strangers.

Spiritual Health

Spiritual health for most people is arguably based on a common inclination towards something greater, someone, or something to whom we can surrender. A dimension, perhaps, away from judgement, sorrow, rationality, and logic. Spiritual health can be defined as the state where one can clock their maximum potential while driven by the meaning and purpose of life and feel happiness within (Dhar, Chaturvedi, and Nandan 2011, 275–82).

In my opinion, people do not consider spiritual health one of the dimensions of health because it is not vital for human survival and we can live without it. However, humans have a fundamental hunger for it. Spirituality can be manifested in several ways—other than religious practices—such as music, dance, yoga, meditation, pranayama, dharana (mindfulness), poetry, etc.

That said, I strongly believe that religion and spirituality hold different meanings. Spirituality is a quest for who we are, why we are born, our fundamental duties towards nature, the purpose of life, etc. Often, this hunger for spirituality leads us to religion. For some, they keep searching for the answers until they find something that resonates with them. When people discover practices that align with their spiritual energies, they experience improved health.

Yogic Transcendental Health

Unlike contemporary definitions, the concept of health according to Ayurvedic and yogic scriptures is broad. It encompasses physical, mental, spiritual, social, and metaphysical aspects of health. To clarify, the transcendental aspects of yoga are being reviewed by the scientific community. Perhaps soon, we will be able to understand these aspects from a contemporary perspective, and they may no longer be considered metaphysical. However, I mean no offence to anyone. In a shloka written around 600 BCE in the Sushrut Samhita, health is defined as:

Sama Dosha Sama Agnischa Sama Dhatu Mala Kriyaaha |
Prasanna Atma Indriya Manaha Swastha Iti Abhidheeyate ||

According to this shloka, we require balanced Tri-Doshas (*Vata, Pitta,* and *Kapha*), digestive fire (*Jatharagni*), metabolism, balanced Dhatus, bacteria, and the proper elimination of waste, along with a happy soul, senses, and mind.

The Three Bodies (*Tri-Sharira*)

The concept of *tri-sharira* or *sharira trya* comes from yogic philosophies. Well-being is the virtue of these three bodies. Yoga does not consider physical fitness as the only criterion. Therefore, we must balance these three bodies. *sharira trya* are:

a. *Sthula Sharira* (the gross or macro body)—made of food and air
b. *Sukshma Sharira* (the subtle or micro body)—made of cognition, behaviour, emotions, etc.
c. *Karana Sharira* (the causal or astral body)—made of subtle seeds that can stem into anything.

The Three Humours (*Tri-Dosha*)

Vata, Pitta, and Kapha are the *tri-doshas*, and all three of them have distinguishable properties. They play a vital role in forming the mental, physical, and social state of an individual. They are often described as the *prakriti* or nature of a being. It is to be noted that people can have combinational prakriti as well where one *dosha* dominates.

a. Vata: It is a combination of *Vayu* (air) and *Akash* (space), responsible for movement and all nervous system activities in the body. People with dominant Vata exhibit these characteristics: Dry skin, tend to speak quickly, fast metabolism, typically have a lean body, are restless, and prefer a hot environment.

b. **Pitta:** It is a combination of *Agni* (fire) and *Jal* (water), governing metabolism, digestion, and transformation in the body and mind. People with a dominant Pitta have the following traits: Oily skin, active, detail-oriented, adaptive, intelligent, medium built, and short-tempered.

c. **Kapha:** It is a combination of *Prithvi* (earth) and *Jal* (water), responsible for structure, stability, and lubrication in the body. People with a dominant Kapha exhibit the following characteristics: Moist skin, slow, calm, weight gain tendencies, soft, fun-loving, and caring.

Three Fundamental Qualities *(Tri-Gunas)*

The concept of *gunas* originates from the Samkhya Philosophy. *Tri-gunas* are three properties of a being, described as Sattva, Rajas, and Tamas. These qualities are believed to be present inside everyone but in different proportions. Therefore, one dominates the others.

1. **Sattva:** It is characterised by calmness, adaptability, goodness, serene tendencies, and balanced sensory temptations.
2. **Rajas:** It is characterised by being active, agile, passionate, exhibiting royal tendencies, and driven by sensory temptations.
3. **Tamas:** It is characterised by inactivity, laziness, denial, procrastination, and less susceptibility to sensory temptations.

The Five Elements (*Pancha Mahabhuta* or *Pancha Tattva*)

Pancha mahabhuta or *pancha tattva* are the five elements through which every species is said to be made. These five elements are *Jal* (water), *Prithvi* (earth), *Agni* (fire), *Vayu* (air), and *Akash* (ether/space). It is believed that our bodies have absorbed everything from the environment. Thus, it is believed that our bodies are composed of:

- 72 per cent of the body is water
- 12 per cent of the body is earth
- 4 per cent of the body is fire
- 6 per cent of the body is air
- 6 per cent of the body is space

The Five Sheaths (*Pancha Kosha*)

The Taittiriya Upanishad (6th century BCE) talks about the five sheaths in detail through the following shloka:

Annam Praanah Manah Buddhih Anandah Iti Panca Te |
Koshastairavrittah Swatma, Vishmritya Sansrutin ||

These are the layers within which our *atman* (spirit) resides:

a. Annamaya Kosha (physical body)—made of food
b. Pranamaya Kosha (energy/breath body)—made of breath & energy
c. Manomaya Kosha (mental body)—made of thoughts, feelings, emotions, and behaviour

d. Vijnanamaya Kosha (intellectual body)—made of wisdom, intuition

e.. Anandamaya Kosha (Bliss body)—made of bliss

The Integration of Yoga and Contemporary Medicine Concerning Health

Modern medicine and the yogic ecosystem offer sophisticated approaches to overall health, with some overlaps and key differences. While modern medicine emphasises physical, mental, and social well-being, the yogic ecosystem introduces additional dimensions. Despite the wide acknowledgement of yoga's effectiveness, some aspects are still poorly understood. Unlike modern medicine, which typically focuses on treating specific issues, the yogic ecosystem aims at a broader goal—enabling individuals to live for 100 years (*Shatayu*). To achieve this, it divides life into four stages, each lasting 25 years, with suggested lifestyle practices for each phase. In contrast, contemporary medical practices tend to address problems more specifically, on a case-by-case basis. For instance, in the case of knee osteoarthritis, modern medicine may focus primarily on the knee joint, while yoga could also address associated muscles, release fascia, relieve stress, and aid rehabilitation. In conclusion, these two approaches are complementary, and, together, they can enhance health and improve quality of life.

5
Health and Safety in Your Yoga Practice: Key Considerations

Everyone is unique, with distinguishable DNA, and what suits one person may not be suitable for another. There are times when we need to accept and choose what works for us best. Trying to force something to work when it isn't designed for us can lead to undesirable outcomes. Unlike many exercise regimes, which may be enjoyable in their way but lack customisability, yoga practices can be adapted to meet our individual needs. However, there are instances when certain yoga practices should be avoided by specific groups of people. In this segment, we will discuss some generalised contraindications to help determine when to practise yoga and when not to.

Note: These are very generalised contraindications. Those with pre-existing conditions or injuries should consult a doctor before attempting Yoga. Additionally, it is advisable to undergo a complete medical check-up before engaging in any form of exercise. This chapter only discusses the most prominent contraindications. There are also numerous other situations where yoga should either be avoided or personalised.

Hernia

A hernia is a condition where an internal part or organ protrudes due to a tear in the surrounding muscles or tissues, typically occurring in the abdominal area. It is important to note that a hernia is not a disease but a surgical condition. In cases of hernia, avoid any yoga pose that puts pressure on the abdominal area. Immediate medical attention may be required.

Heart Ailments

For heart conditions, consulting a qualified doctor is essential. There are several types of heart ailments, each with specific requirements. However, as a general guideline, people with heart conditions should avoid sudden, flow-based yoga practices or those that cause the heart rate to rise excessively. Building a practice gradually is advisable.

Osteoarthritis

What we commonly refer to as arthritis is often a specific type known as osteoarthritis. Osteoarthritis is a widespread condition, characterised by the wear and tear of the joint cartilage. The absence of this cushioning mechanism results in pain caused by friction between bones. Osteoarthritis can affect any joint, and in such cases, yoga practice should be modified to avoid putting strain on the affected joints.

Rheumatoid Arthritis

Rheumatoid arthritis is an inflammatory and autoimmune condition where the body's immune system attacks the tissues of the joints. Yoga is often beneficial for those with rheumatoid arthritis and can be considered an adjunct therapy (Telles and Singh 2012, 81). However, when the condition worsens, a low-impact yoga session is more suitable.

Carpal Tunnel Syndrome (CTS)

Carpal tunnel syndrome is characterised by numbness or tingling in the fingers or hands due to a pinched nerve in the wrist joints. In such cases, yoga practitioners should avoid placing too much strain on the wrist joints. Additionally, they should refrain from excessive upward and downward motion of the hands and postures that require gripping.

Joint Injuries

Joint injuries, such as bursitis, tendonitis, sprains, or osteoporosis, can occur for various reasons. Before attempting yoga, it is critical to understand the type of injury and proceed accordingly.

Spinal Injuries

Spinal injuries can be a serious concern, often caused by ageing, motor vehicle accidents, sports injuries, or wear and tear. Certain yoga postures should be avoided or modified to suit individual needs in cases of spinal injury.

Pregnancy

Pregnancy is a delicate period, usually divided into three trimesters. The first trimester is considered the most delicate, with most miscarriages occurring during this time. The second trimester is relatively safer, though caution is still advised, while in the third trimester, women may be more prone to overextending themselves, which should be avoided. Prenatal and postnatal yoga sessions should be carefully planned.

Menstruation

During menstruation, the lining of the uterus sheds when a fertilised egg is not implanted. It is believed that inverted poses (upside-down asanas) can cause discomfort. Avoid inverted asanas, core-strengthening poses, deep forward bends, and deep backbends during menstruation. Asanas to avoid include Sirsasana (Headstand), Sarvangasana (Shoulder Stand), Viparita Karani (Inverted Pose), Navasana (Boat Pose),

Dhanurasana (Bow Pose), and Uttanasana (Standing Forward Bend), among others.

Recent Surgery

Yoga after surgery requires careful consideration and personalised guidance. While avoiding strenuous practices is generally recommended initially, gentle movements and breathing exercises may be appropriate depending on the type of surgery, recovery stage, and medical advice. It's important to consult with your doctor to explore safe and supportive yoga practices that can aid in recovery.

Glaucoma

Certain yoga postures increase intraocular pressure, which can strain the eyes. Most of these are inverted poses. Individuals with glaucoma should avoid such asanas.

Diabetes

In diabetes, it is essential to consult with a doctor before starting yoga. Together, you can create a personalised plan that considers the type and severity of diabetes, your medication regimen, and individual needs.

These are some of the common contraindications one should keep in mind before attempting any yoga practice. Throughout this book, a variety of modifications for each yoga pose have been added, which can be used in some conditions. However, if you have specific contraindications or conditions, consult a doctor and practise yoga under the guidance of a professional. Kindly remember that almost all books cannot substitute professional advice.

6

Exploring the Basics of Yoga Alignment

Yoga is about uniting the body, mind, and beyond. To maximise the benefits, you need to follow precise cues. Difficulties with the cues or movements can break the spirit of the practice, as they divert the practitioner's attention. In anatomical terms—cues, the GPS of yoga—pinpoint movements and limb positioning that not only minimise distractions but also ease the flow, safeguard the joints, effectively engage muscles, and facilitate efficient movement.

Directional Anatomical Terms

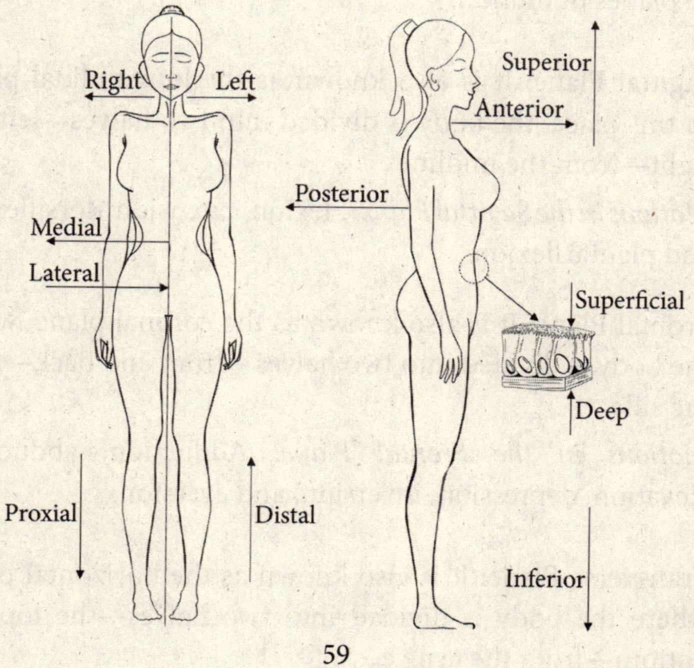

- Anterior: Located in the front
- Posterior: Located in the rear
- Medial: Located towards the midline
- Lateral: Located away from the midline
- Superior: Located above
- Inferior: Located below
- Superficial: Close to the surface
- Deep: Under/beneath the surface
- Proximal: Close to the attachment point
- Distal: Away from the attachment point

Planes of Motion

The planes of motion are valuable for depicting and assessing movement. When a specific movement is mentioned in relation to the planes of motion, researchers can evaluate the direction and extent of motion in joints and body segments. There are three planes of motion:

Sagittal Plane: It is also known as the longitudinal plane. In this place, the body is divided into two halves—left and right—from the midline.

Motions in the Sagittal Plane: Flexion, extension, dorsiflexion, and plantarflexion.

Frontal Plane: It is also known as the coronal plane, where the body is divided into two halves—front and back—from the side.

Motions in the Frontal Plane: Adduction, abduction, elevation, depression, inversion, and eversion.

Transverse Plane: It is also known as the horizontal plane, where the body is divided into two halves—the top and bottom—from the centre.

Motions in the Transverse Plane: Rotation, internal rotation, external rotation, pronation, supination, circumduction, horizontal flexion (adduction), and horizontal extension (abduction).

Movement-Oriented Anatomical Terms

Flexion: A bending movement where the joint angle decreases from the standard anatomical position. Like, bending the elbows or knees or bending the spine forward.

Extension: The straightening movement where the angle between the body parts (joints) increases. For instance, straightening the elbows and knees.

Hyperextension: It refers to the movement of a joint beyond the standard anatomical position. Examples: Bending the elbows or knees past their normal range or the leg moving backwards beyond a standing position.

Abduction: The movement where our joints move away from the midline of the body. Like, raising the arms or legs sideways.

Adduction: The movement where our joints return to the midline. Examples: Bringing the arms or legs back down to the side from an abducted position.

Protrusion: The forward movement of a joint or structure. For instance, protracting the shoulder blades or the forward movement of the neck.

Retrusion: The backward movement of a joint or structure. Examples: Retracting the shoulder blades, pulling them towards the spine, or pulling the lower jaw back.

Elevation: The movement where the joints move superiorly or upwards. For example, lifting the shoulders towards the ears and elevating the jaw while biting or chewing.

Depression: The movement where the joints move inferiorly or downwards. Example: lowering the shoulders back to a neutral position, bringing them down when relaxing the upper body or depressing the jaw when opening the mouth.

Rotation: The movement where the joint moves around its axis. Examples: Rotating fingers, shoulder joints, hip joints, or knee joints.

There are two types of rotations:

a. Medial (internal) rotation: Rotating a limb towards the midline—turning the head from side to side or rotating the arm inwards.
b. Lateral (external) rotation: Rotating a limb away from the midline—rotating the arm or leg outwards.

Circumduction: It is the circular movement where the limb (joint) moves along its long axis, combining flexion, extension, abduction, and adduction. Example: Circularly moving the arm, shoulders and hip joints.

Supination: The movement where the palms face up. For instance, turning the hand so the palm faces the sky.

Pronation: The movement where the palms face down. Example: Turning the hand so the palm faces the floor.

Plantar Flexion: The movement where the foot moves away from the anterior shin bone. Like, standing on your toes.

Dorsiflexion: The movement where the foot moves towards the anterior shin bone. Like, standing on your heels.

Inversion: Turning the sole of the foot inwards, toward the midline. For instance, standing on the outer edge of your foot.

Eversion: Turning the sole of the foot outwards, away from the midline. For instance, standing on the inner edge of your foot.

Ipsilateral: It is the same side of the body where the motion occurs. For example, if you bend to the right side, in a triangle pose, that side becomes ipsilateral.

Contralateral: It is the opposite side of the body where the motion occurs. For instance, if you bend to the right side in a triangle pose, the left side becomes contralateral.

Pelvic Tilts

The movement of the pelvis in relation to the spine is referred to as pelvic tilt. This movement can be either an anterior tilt (forward tilt) or a posterior tilt (backward tilt). Understanding pelvic tilts is crucial for maintaining proper posture, spinal alignment, and overall core stability.

> Anterior Pelvic Tilt: The movement of the pelvis where it rotates forward. The anterior pelvic tilt is typically accompanied by an arched or erect back.
>
> Posterior Pelvic Tilt: The movement of the pelvis where it rotates backwards. The posterior pelvic tilt is typically accompanied by a flat or curved spine.

The Importance of Learning these Terminologies

Learning these terminologies will help you understand every physical movement better, not just asanas. It's akin to developing an X-ray vision that can track every movement, joint action, and muscle that forms these movements, which enables smoother personalisation. For example, individuals who walk with their toes pointing outwards, also known as duck feet or out-toeing, may exhibit noticeable misalignments, suggesting that stretching the hamstring and gluteal muscles could be beneficial. However, figuring out what works and when requires a gradual learning curve. In the upcoming chapters, I have mentioned asanas with joint action and muscles associated to make learning convenient.

7
Exploring the Connection between Yoga and Organ Systems

Have you wondered how yoga, an ancient tradition, impacts our organ systems under the scrutiny of contemporary science? Humanity has longed for a healthy life, leading us to the scientific exploration of living organisms, known as biomedical science. This has significantly magnified our understanding of anatomy and physiology. As a result, it has led to the rigorous testing of various practices, including yoga, through the lens of organ and organ systems. Yoga is a tradition over 5,000 years old, and, therefore, there was scepticism about whether it aligns well with contemporary science.

Spoiler—contemporary science considers yoga the best friend of our holistic health. In this chapter, we will explore how yoga, with easy-to-do asanas, has a profound impact on our cardiovascular health, spine, muscles, nervous system, hormonal balance, and much more.

From Cells to Organ Systems: Building the Body

Did you know that yoga can help slow down senescence? A study (Tolahunase et al., 2017), published in a reputable journal, concluded that yoga and meditation help improve biomarkers of cellular ageing. A cell is the smallest functional unit of a living body. It is also known as the building block of the body, and we are a union (yoga) of trillions of cells. If we rewind time by a few million years, all aquatic and terrestrial life forms were once unicellular, meaning, they were made of only one cell. Through the process of evolution, life became multicellular. Our cells still function independently, though in tandem with each other.

Later, the functionally identical cells formed specialised groups, called tissues. Biomedical science divides tissues into four groups—epithelial, muscular, nervous, and connective. Permutations and combinations of these tissues form an organ. Most organs comprise all four types of tissues—for instance, the stomach. Finally, systematically orchestrated organs form an organ system. We will now learn about yoga and its profound impact on various organ systems.

Bio-Individuality

Is every yoga asana suitable for everyone? The concept of bio-individuality is instrumental in explaining how one's anatomy and physiology can differ from others. We each have a distinct body that digests, perceives, and manages things differently. Bio-individuality is often discussed from a nutritional point of view. However, yoga can also benefit from this concept.

We know that each body is anatomically unique, meaning, generic steps may or may not work for everyone. Some examples of bio-individuality are obvious, such as lordosis (arched back), kyphosis (swayback), knock knees (genu valgum), and bow legs (genu varum). Whether it's a subtle difference or an obvious one, the degree of movement during an asana is bound to vary. Therefore, it makes sense to personalise asanas as much as possible to suit individuals correctly.

The Integumentary System

The integumentary system is the body's outer covering, serving as the first line of defence. It protects our body from the external environment and allows us to sense pressure, temperature, touch, and motion.

Skin, Yoga, and Glowing Skin

I have met several people who believe that yogis and gurus have exceptionally healthy and radiant skin, irrespective of their complexion. Fortunately, for them, current evidence supports this belief. In one study, it was found that yoga and meditation are low-risk solutions that can be integrated into therapy to treat several dermatological (skin-related) conditions, including atopic dermatitis, psoriasis, self-induced skin conditions, and others (Graubard et al., 2021). So, now you know how to save a lot on cosmetics.

The Skeletal System

If you struggle with hamstring stretches and backbends, it could be due to an uncomfortable pelvis. Similarly, discomfort in Gomukhasana (Cow Face Pose) could stem from an uncomfortable position of the scapula. Understanding these aspects of the skeletal system can enhance your yoga practice and overall body mechanics. The skeletal system provides a structural framework, protection, shock absorption, movement, and more. Contrary to common perception, the skeletal system is quite lively. Beyond its seemingly brittle structure, it is dynamic—maintaining and renewing itself, producing blood cells, and storing and releasing minerals. Apart from bones, the skeletal system includes three slightly more flexible components—cartilage, ligaments, and tendons. The skeletal system is divided into two parts: Axial (80 bones) and appendicular (126 bones).

Bones, Yoga, and Bone Density

Bones are tough and have high tensile strength, yet they are not entirely brittle. They appear pinkish-white and constantly undergo several processes, including the production of blood cells, repair, and renewal. When challenged by yoga, particularly weight-bearing asanas (Warrior I Pose or Chair Pose) and dynamic practices such as Sukshma Vyayama (yogic push-ups, yogic squats, etc.) and vinyasa, bone density increases (Fernández et al., 2021).

Cartilage, Yoga, and Joint Health

In the yoga community, practitioners often claim to have better joint health. While their claims may sound dubious to non-practitioners, studies prove that yoga promotes joint health. Cartilage, which is slightly more delicate than bones, supports the bones. However, it has poor regenerative powers as it lacks blood vessels. It depends on the diffusion mechanism for nutrition absorption, which relies on movement.

Yoga promotes joint health by mobilising our joints in all possible directions, providing nutrition and preventing damage to the cartilage. For instance, the knee joint can easily be mobilised by asanas such as Ustrasana (Camel Pose—flexion of the knee joint), Paschimottanasana (Seated Forward Bend Pose—extension of the knee joint), and Vajrasana (Thunderbolt Pose—slight rotation of the knee joint). These movements adequately spread nutrients to the surrounding cartilage while maintaining a sufficient range of motion. Additionally, yoga also helps with degenerated cartilage. Osteoarthritis, a common disorder in older adults, is caused by wear and tear of the cartilage. Yoga, with good evidence, is known to diminish pain and improve overall quality of life in osteoarthritis (Kan et al., 2016).

Ligaments, Yoga, and the Range of Motion

The degree to which we can move a joint is known as its range of motion. Studies have concluded that yoga enhances our flexibility and range of motion (Polsgrove et al., 2016). It is worth noting that a diminished range of motion is often linked with tight ligaments. Ligaments are tough, fibrous connective tissues that connect one bone to another at a joint. If ligaments are optimally 'loose', they increase our range of motion.

Tendons, Yoga, and Injury Prevention

Have you noticed a slightly moveable structure right above your heels? It is not a bone, but a strong tendon called the Achilles tendon. Like all tendons, the Achilles is invaluable for movement, including yoga. Tendons connect muscles to bones. They are dense, fibrous connective tissues designed to withstand pulls and strains. The tendon hosts the Golgi tendon organ (GTO), a mechanoreceptor that detects tension and prevents injuries. For instance, when we assume Uttanasana (Standing Forward Bend Pose), GTOs can detect tension and may initiate temporary relaxation in the hamstring muscles to protect against any damage to the tendon and muscle complex. This may translate to more hamstring stretch. However, pushing GTOs too much can result in injury.

Joints, Yoga, and Injury Prevention

Lately, yoga has been encouraged by physiotherapists for sports injury rehabilitation. Most injuries affect our joints, therefore, understanding joint mechanics is pivotal in preventing injuries. A joint is the junction where two or more bones come together. Apart from bones, cartilage, ligaments, and tendons also participate in various joints. Based on movement and structure, joints are categorised into three types: Fibrous joints (immovable), cartilaginous joints (slightly movable), and synovial joints (movable). Synovial joints, the most abundant type, are the most relevant from a yogic perspective.

Synovial joints have a joint capsule containing synovial fluid. This fluid—a natural lubricant—minimises friction between two bones and makes the joint mobile. Any damage to synovial fluid can induce pain. Yoga is proven to slow down the deterioration of synovial fluid volume (Singh et al., 2018), thereby minimising contact between two rough bones and contributing to prolonged joint health. Additionally, like other exercise regimes, yoga also strengthens our muscles. Stronger muscles help stabilise joints, preventing injuries.

The Spine, Yoga, and Spinal Health

The evolution of the spine was significant in enabling vertebrates to have swift movement and better coordination. Interestingly, while walking, we rely more on the movement of our spine than the hip joint. The spine protects the spinal cord and consists of 26 vertebrae. It is divided into five segments—the cervical spine (seven bones), the thoracic spine (12 bones), the lumbar spine (five bones), the sacrum (one bone), and the coccyx (one bone). The thoracic spine offers greater rotation but minimal flexion and extension, whereas the sacral (sacrum and coccyx) region offers negligible movement. Conversely, the cervical and lumbar regions are mobile and offer a wide range of motion. However, with great mobility comes the risk of injury.

Yoga can be a great way to keep the spine healthy and active. The spinal discs are prone to injury for various reasons, including wear and tear, ageing, acute injury, sedentary lifestyle, and prolonged incorrect posture. The spinal discs receive nutrients through imbibition, a process that relies on movement. Yoga is beneficial in this regard as it mobilises the spine in every possible direction through asanas such as Vakrasana (Twisted Pose), Salamba Bhujangasana (Sphinx Pose), Tiryaka Tadasana (Swaying Palm Tree Pose), Cat and Cow mobility, etc. Thus, yoga helps keep spinal discs healthy and increases flexibility (Grabara, 2016). Furthermore, yoga helps prevent low back pain, a common spinal disorder (Cramer, et al., 2013).

The Muscular System

Ask yourself, if not for aesthetics, what does your muscular system offer? Why should you train it?

Beyond aesthetics, our muscular system has transformational powers. It is an instrumental system concerned with muscles and their motion. Furthermore, it is influential in the stabilisation of joints, heat production, digestion, and much more.

Muscles, Yoga, and Agility

Muscles are specialised tissues containing ample blood supply. They contract, sustain motion, and change shape. However, they do only one thing—pull or contract. There are three types of muscles—smooth muscles that form the walls of various organs, cardiac muscles that form the walls of the heart, and skeletal muscles that allow various movements. Imagine our muscles as sponge balls that contract, produce force, and retain shape.

Type of contractions:

- Isotonic contraction: Contraction of the muscle while the muscle length is subject to change
- Concentric contraction: Also known as the shortening contraction where the muscle length decreases

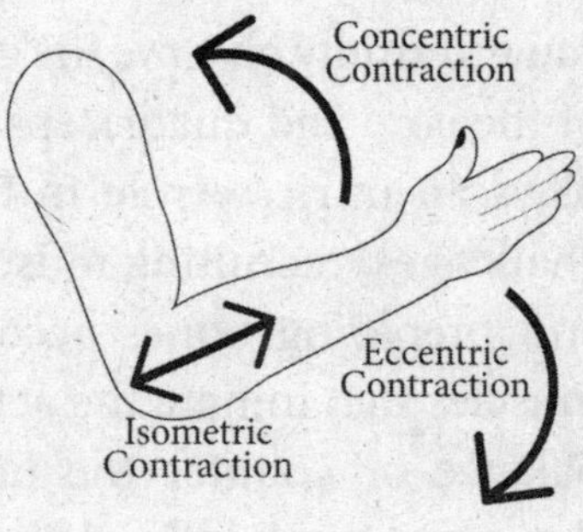

- Eccentric contraction: It is a lengthening contraction where the muscle length increases while resisting greater force
- Isometric contraction: Contraction of a muscle while the muscle length remains unchanged

Most asanas are based on isometric contractions. However, a typical yoga session involves all three types of contractions. It is because a typical yoga session includes Surya Namaskar (Sun Salutations), Sukshma Vyayama (pre-practices/warm-ups/dynamic mobility practices), asanas, and more. Furthermore, most yoga sessions involve flow-based movements, where one moves into a peak pose and then transitions out of it. During these stages, our muscles undergo all sorts of contractions. Overall, when practising yoga, our muscles perform mobility, endurance, contractibility, elasticity, muscle coordination, and beyond (Tran et al., 2001).

Understanding Contractions

The contemporary world is fascinated by the power of our muscles, and rightly so. Our muscles are in feedback loops with the nervous system, adapting physiologically to meet challenges. Yoga effectively integrates muscle contraction to its advantage. Just before we perform Navasana (Boat Pose), we can mindfully observe the gradual recruitment and contraction of the core and quadriceps muscles. Thus, the nervous system plays an intricate role in formulating contractions, assessing challenges, recruiting muscles, enhancing neural connections, and preparing bones accordingly. Based on movement, the muscles that initiate the actions are called 'agonists', those that balance or counter the motion are called 'antagonists', and those that work in tandem with agonists are called 'synergists'.

In Navasana (Boat Pose), agonists are core and quadriceps muscles, antagonists are spinal and hamstring muscles, and synergists are the pectoral and adductor muscles.

Types of Contraction Mechanisms

While various asanas appear strikingly symmetrical, their muscle contraction mechanisms differ significantly. There are primarily three types of contraction mechanisms that function in various yoga practices, depending on the type of movement. For instance, in Adho Mukha Svanasana (Downward-Facing Dog Pose), the quadriceps muscles (agonists) contract, causing the hamstring muscles (antagonist) to relax. This is an example of reciprocal inhibition. According to the law of reciprocal inhibition, when one muscle contracts, the opposing muscles relax.

However, in Adho Mukha Vrksasana (Handstand Pose), the mechanism is different. The core muscles, deltoids, and other muscles around the shoulder and scapula contract simultaneously to maintain the position. This is an example of co-contraction.

Likewise, there exists a third mechanism called autogenic inhibition, which relaxes muscles when excessive strain is applied to the muscle-tendon (Golgi tendon) organ to prevent injuries. For instance, in Ardha Matsyendrasana (Half Lord of the Fishes Pose), the body is in deep trunk rotation, which induces significant strain on the spinal and abdominal muscles, the Golgi tendon organ detects this tension and triggers the release of these muscles.

Prime Muscles in the Human Body

Our body is comprised of over 600 muscles. Most of these muscles play a vital role in the formulation of movements, heat production, etc. However, some muscles are larger, stronger, and much more significant than others. Here are some prime muscles that are vital for yoga as well as other activities.

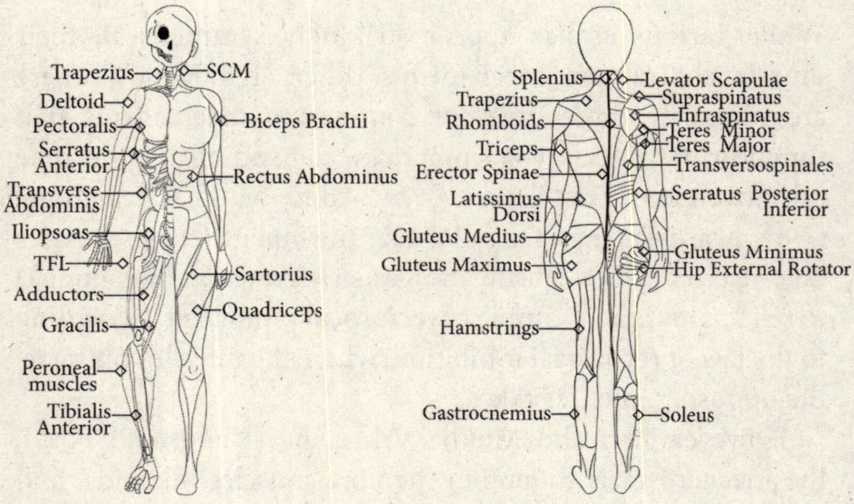

- Head (Skull)
  - Masseter
- The neck (cervical spine)
  - Sternocleidomastoid, longus (Colli and Capitis), splenius, and upper trapezius
- Upper limbs
  - Deltoid, biceps brachii, triceps brachii, wrist pronators, and wrist supinators
  - Rotator cuff (supraspinatus, infraspinatus, teres minor, and subscapularis—SITS)

- Trunk
    - o Pectoralis major and minor, rhomboid, serratus anterior, trapezius, quadratus lumborum, and latissimus dorsi
- The spine
    - o The erector spinae group (longissimus, iliocostalis, and spinalis) and transversospinalis (semispinalis, multifidus, and rotatores)
- The core
    - o Rectus abdominis, external and internal obliques, and transverse abdominis
- The lower limbs
    - o Hips
- Gluteal group (maximus, medius, and minimus), iliopsoas, hip external rotator group (piriformis, gemellus, and obturator internus), and tensor fascia lata (TFL)
    - o Pelvic floor muscles
    - o Levator ani and coccygeus
- Thighs
    - o Quadriceps group (rectus femoris, vastus—lateralis, intermedius, and medialis),
    - o Hamstring group (biceps femoris, semitendinosus, semimembranosus)
    - o Adductor group (adductor magnus, longus, brevis, and minimus), gracilis, and sartorius

- Lower Legs
    - Gastrocnemius soleus, tibialis anterior and posterior, and fibularis or peroneus (longus and brevis)

The Nervous System

Cognitive abilities, thoughts, creativity, improvisation, and inventions stem from the nervous system. This intricate system interacts with the internal body and external environment. It is divided into two parts—the central nervous system (CNS) and the peripheral nervous system (PNS). The CNS is primarily composed of the brain and spinal cord. Whereas, the PNS extends to the remaining body and is composed of the somatic nervous system (SNS), the enteric nervous system (ENS), and the autonomic nervous system (ANS). The SNS is responsible for conscious action (voluntary), reflexes, and relaying sensory signals, such as regulated breathing (pranayama), movement (asana), rapid blinking of eyes, etc. Conversely, the ANS automates our essential tasks and cannot be consciously controlled (involuntary), such as digestion, respiration, circulation, etc.

Did you know you have a second brain in the body? It's called the ENS and is located in the gut. It hosts several neurons that can act semi-independently. It regulates motility, digestion, secretion, peristalsis (a series of involuntary muscle contractions that move food and fluids through the digestive system), and more. The nervous system is closely linked—if one part of the nervous system is affected, it cascades to the rest.

Autonomic Nervous System, Yoga, and Unwinding

Can we unwind with yoga? Let's find out the underlying science. The ANS is divided into two parts—the Sympathetic Nervous System (SNS) and the Parasympathetic Nervous System (PNS). The SNS is also known as the 'stress response' or the 'fight or flight' response. To imagine its functions appropriately, think of being chased by a tiger. To survive, you will need increased respiration, higher heart rate, faster circulation, more glucose, quick muscle movement, and no digestion because survival comes first. On the contrary, the PNS is the 'peacetime response' or the 'rest and digest' response. To imagine its functions correctly, picture yourself on a stress-free vacation. To enjoy your time, you will require relaxed respiration, heart rate, circulation, less glucose, relaxed muscles, and proper digestion.

Both systems coexist and are vital for our survival; however, imbalances can be serious. For your information, the imbalances in the ANS often result in stress, anxiety, and depression. Studies have shown that yoga helps to balance the ANS with the help of two mechanisms—downregulating the SNS response by practising dynamic yogic practices, including vinyasa, hatha yoga, and surya namaskar, and upregulating the PNS response through serene yogic practices, including pranayama, meditation, and yoga nidra.

Brain, Yoga, and Improved Cognitive Abilities

Our intelligence is determined by our cognitive abilities. The brain processes information, relays motor signals to form movements, and accepts sensory signals to maintain homeostasis (an optimal healthy state). However, the brain is divided into several centres, out of which a few of them are known to diminish cognitive output when overactive. Yoga can be an apt way to downregulate these centres, enhancing cognitive production. A systematic review involving mostly asanas concluded a positive correlation between yoga and brain health (Gothe et al., 2019). This study also unearthed yoga's potential to positively influence the brain's anatomy, in turn, signifying that the effects of asanas extend to mental health and are well beyond the physical body.

Neurons, Yoga, and Somatosensation

Yoga nidra, a popular technique among yogis, is the practice where one focuses on the somatosensory (conscious sensory) perception derived from the neurons. They are the smallest functional units of the nervous system and are divided into two types—sensory neurons that receive sensory information and motor neurons that transmit motor information. Neurons are vital for forging our thoughts, feelings, movements, deciphering sensory inputs, and more. Yoga approaches both neurons distinctively. For instance, Pratyahara, the fifth limb of Ashtanga (eight limbs) yoga is directed towards withdrawing our attention from sensory information. Whereas, asanas are directed to act on the neuromuscular junction where motor neurons and muscular tissues join. Studies suggest that physical activities (such as yoga) can cause hypertrophy of neuromuscular junctions and speed up the recovery from peripheral nerve injuries (Nishimune et al., 2014). However, practices like yoga nidra combine these two aspects by being aware of all somatosensory perceptions.

The Circulatory System

Did you know, our blood vessels can wrap the entire earth multiple times? The circulatory system is concerned with the transportation of resources to each cell in the body. To do so, it comprises a heart and a complex network of blood vessels called arteries, veins, and capillaries. Arteries (except pulmonary arteries) carry pure blood, veins (except pulmonary veins) carry impure blood, and tiny capillaries carry gaseous exchange.

Heart, Yoga, and Cardiovascular Endurance

Heart health is constantly making its way into the news but for troubling reasons. Beyond ECG and limited fat intake, moderate weekly cardio exercises including yoga are suggested by doctors.

The heart—the centrepiece of the circulatory system—acts as a mechanical motor (dual pump) that pumps blood. The heart walls are made of cardiac muscles that can withstand tremendous pressure. The heart is divided into four parts—the right atrium and right ventricle carrying oxygen-poor blood, the left atrium and left ventricle carrying oxygen-rich blood. The heart rate, regulated by the ANS, varies depending on the activities. Heart rate variability (HRV) is a way to measure the potency of the heart and ANS, which signifies cardiovascular endurance. Yoga is proven to improve HRV, thus improving cardiovascular endurance (Kuppusamy et al., 2020). Furthermore, yoga is also effective as a preventive measure. Practising asanas, particularly Sarvangasana (Shoulder Stand Pose) and Ardha Halasana (Half Plough Pose) can help prevent cardiovascular diseases (Jayasinghe, 2004).

Blood, Yoga, and Blood Pressure

With 1.28 billion people experiencing high blood pressure, the general awareness needs to be improved. Blood carries red blood cells (RBCs), white blood cells (WBCs), platelets nutrients, minerals, oxygen, waste, etc. RBCs manage the transportation, WBCs fight invaders, and platelets prevent blood loss. The amount of pressure exerted by our blood on the walls of the arteries is known as blood pressure. The urinary system with hormonal inputs from the adrenal gland influences our blood pressure. Typically, it stays around 120/80 mmHg in a healthy person. However, increased blood pressure is known as hypertension or high blood pressure. Enough evidence suggests that asanas and other limbs of yoga can be added as a complementary therapy for managing high blood pressure (Cramer et al., 2014).

The Respiratory System

The respiratory system is responsible for gas exchange. Air follows a sequential path through the nose, nasal cavity, pharynx, larynx, trachea, bronchi, bronchioles, and finally the alveoli. The alveoli are tiny sacs where the final gas exchange takes place. The respiratory system also has secondary functions, such as enabling the sense of smell through nasal receptors, facilitating voice formulation (phonation) via the larynx, and humidifying air through the sinuses.

Breath, Yoga, and the Power of the Diaphragm

How do we breathe? Have you noticed your belly expanding during inhalation? What is diaphragmatic breathing, let's find out. Breathing involves a crucial muscle called the diaphragm, which separates the respiratory system from the digestive system. When we take a deep breath, the diaphragm contracts and moves downward, causing the belly to inflate. Inhalation occurs as the diaphragm contracts and accessory muscles of respiration (such as the sternocleidomastoid, pectoralis, trapezius, intercostals, and abdominals) lift the ribcage, allowing the lungs to expand. This creates lower pressure inside the lungs compared to the outside environment, causing air to flow in. The reverse process leads to exhalation.

The diaphragm works in feedback with the brain's respiratory centres. Fortunately, it can be controlled both voluntarily and involuntarily. Pranayama practices can influence breathing and, by extension, the diaphragm. Techniques like Dirgha Svasana (Three-Part Breath), belly breathing (diaphragmatic breathing), and Bhramari pranayama (Humming Bee Breath) can help regulate the nervous system, leading to a calm mind, balanced metabolism, better emotional regulation, and more.

The Endocrine System

The endocrine system consists of hormone-secreting glands linked through feedback loops in the bloodstream. It complements the nervous system by producing long-term effects in the body, regulating stress responses, metabolism, growth, and mineral balance while maintaining homeostasis (an optimal internal environment).

- *Hypothalamus*: A key link between the nervous and endocrine systems
- *Pituitary gland*: The master gland, influencing the endocrine system via a variety of hormones
- *Pineal gland*: Regulates the sleep-wake cycle (circadian rhythm)
- *Thyroid gland*: Controls energy use (metabolism) and calcium homeostasis
- *Parathyroid glands*: Help maintain calcium balance
- *Thymus gland*: Trains T-lymphocytes, a part of the immune system
- *Islets of Langerhans in the pancreas*: Regulate blood glucose
- *Adrenal glands*: Produce essential hormones like cortisol, adrenaline, and noradrenaline
- *Testes*: Secrete male hormones
- *Ovaries*: Secrete female hormones

HPA Axis, Yoga, and Stress

Our stress response often works against us. To maintain allostasis (a stable body amid physiological changes), the hypothalamus, pituitary, and adrenal glands form the HPA axis. The HPA axis and sympathetic nervous system (SNS) respond similarly to both physical and mental stressors. Overactivation of the HPA axis leads to rapid breathing, irregular heartbeat, higher blood glucose, disrupted digestion, poor sleep, and impaired brain reward pathways. Chronic mental stress can contribute to conditions like type 2 diabetes, obesity, and cardiovascular disease. To counter this, practising Surya Namaskar and asanas can help regulate the HPA axis. Surya Namaskar can influence the hypothalamus and lower cortisol (the stress hormone), providing a way to unwind and relax (Agre et al., 2021).

Cortisol, Yoga, and Weight Loss

Could stress be the reason for weight gain rather than poor dietary habits? Cortisol, the stress hormone, plays a significant role. Activation of the HPA axis increases cortisol, which, in turn, raises glucose levels in the body. When glucose is abundant, fat is not utilised, leading to increased fat storage. Thus, stress may contribute more to weight gain than poor eating habits. To break this cycle, practising Kapalabhati (Skull Shining Breath), Surya Namaskar, and asanas can help reduce stress, lower cortisol, and support weight management (Thirthalli et al., 2013). Yoga may improve sleep, reduce stress hormones like cortisol, and restore the body's natural balance.

The Digestive System

The digestive system is the largest organ system, which is responsible for the absorption of food vitamins, minerals, and nutrients by our cells. It breaks down the food through chemical and mechanical processes. Sensory inputs from smell, sight, and taste mark the onset of digestion. The teeth break food mechanically, the tongue stirs it, and the pharynx—along with the oesophagus—transports it to the stomach. The stomach digests food (bolus) through gastric secretions. The food (chyme) enters the duodenum of the small intestine, where bile juice from the liver and pancreatic juice from the pancreas are released through a common pipe (ampulla of Vater). From here, nutrients, minerals, and water are absorbed into the small intestine. The large intestine absorbs minimal water and stores the stool in the rectum, which is ultimately defecated via the anus. A series of simultaneous contractions, called peristalsis, gradually push the food forward in the digestive canal, called the gastrointestinal tract (GI tract).

Gut, Yoga, and Yogic Diet

It goes without saying that 'we are what we eat'; however, there's more to it than meets the eye. As discussed earlier, the gut houses the ENS, which hosts several trillion microbiota that aid in our digestion. The composition of microbiota varies greatly depending on the food we consume. Despite being located within the large intestine, small intestine, and stomach, it can influence our mood, cravings, and thoughts. A healthy diet supports a healthy ENS and mood, and vice versa. The functioning of the ENS reminds me of a shloka from the Ayurvedic text Ashtanga Hridayam:

> *Tanmana Bhojangatah Chittah* [8.35]

Meaning, while eating, our thoughts, gratitude, and food impact our psychology and digestion. However, various yogic texts extensively discuss *Mitahara* or a 'balanced diet', where half the stomach is reserved for food, one-quarter for water, and one-quarter is left empty. Additionally, yoga keeps the concept of 'Ahimsa' or 'non-violence' at its core; thus, non-vegetarian food is often discouraged by yogis. A plant-based diet is encouraged instead. Their stance is research-backed—a study revealed that a plant-based diet can help reduce body weight with improved gut microbiota (Verdam et al., 2013).

Moreover, beyond diet, practising Asanas has also been proven effective for digestion as it activates the PNS or the 'rest and digest system' (Paramasivam et al., 2021).

The Lymphatic System

The lymphatic system maintains fluid balance in the body while fighting invaders. To maintain the fluid balance, the lymphatic system drains extracellular fluid and returns it to the circulatory system. Lymphocytes, the prime cells of the lymphatic system, make up about 20 per cent of the total WBCs and are specialised in fighting invaders, pathogens, etc. Lymph, a fluid containing mostly lymphocytes, travels through lymphatic vessels like the blood vessels. Organs producing lymphocytes are called lymphatic organs. Primary lymphatic organs include bone marrow and the thymus gland. Additionally, the spleen, tonsil, and adenoid play key roles in fighting infections. Lastly, lymph nodes help prevent the development of cancer by monitoring and clearing lymph fluid.

Inflammation, Yoga, and Immune System

Inflammation helps us understand how our immune system responds to a threat. It is a mechanism of our immune system and is not necessarily detrimental as it often signals a battle against invaders, healing, and clean-up. However, some inflammations can trigger certain diseases, such as arthritis, diabetes, asthma, fatty liver, autoimmune disorders, cancer, etc. Asanas, such as Adho Mukha Svanasana (Downward Facing Dog pose), Ustrasana (Camel Pose), Bhujangasana (Cobra Pose), and restorative practices help to twist, massage, and compress the entire lymphatic system, thus, clearing the lymphatic drainage. Additionally, yoga has another mechanism where stress modulation enhances immunity.

Hence, Yoga practices also boost our immunity, contributing to reduced inflammation and a better quality of life (Falkenberg et al., 2018).

The Urinary System

Understanding the urinary system can be a way to promote our urinary function and sexual health. The urinary system is responsible for clearing the excess fluid, minerals, ions, and other waste that are soluble in water. Its function begins in the kidneys, the primary organs responsible for filtering blood to remove excess minerals, fluids, and waste. The kidneys transport filtered fluid (urine) to the bladder via the ureters. The urinary bladder, a muscular pouch, temporarily stores urine received from the kidneys. Finally, the urethra, a tube connected to the external genitalia, allows urine to exit the body.

Pelvic Floor Muscles, Yoga, and Orgasm

Is there a way to delay orgasm? Yes! The pelvic floor muscles, acting as hidden hammocks, are located at the base of the pelvis. The levator ani and coccygeus, two major pelvic floor muscles, work in close coordination with the diaphragm. Simply put, these muscles help us control the bladder and bowel movements. Additionally, they can also help delay orgasm. Tight pelvic floor muscles can cause premature orgasms, uncomfortable urgency, and urinary and anal incontinence. Asanas like Utkatasana (Chair Pose), Setu Bandhasana (Bridge Pose), and Malasana (Deep Squat Pose) are suggested to strengthen and release these pelvic floor muscles, improving their function. Stronger pelvic muscles translate to better control over orgasm and urination. This is consistent with current evidence; for instance, yoga has been proven effective for women experiencing urinary incontinence (Kannan et al.,

2022). Furthermore, it may also delay orgasm, leading to better sexual health, as there is a strong link between pelvic floor muscle strength and orgasm (Sartori et al., 2020).

The Reproductive System

The reproductive system is responsible for gender characteristics and the propagation of our species.

Male Reproductive System

Men are facing a catastrophic rise in infertility, and yoga can be a way to prevent further deterioration. The male reproductive system is responsible for male characteristics, hormone production, sperm cell production, and more. The penis, the male external genitalia, releases both sperm and urine via the urethra. The primary reproductive function of the penis is to deliver sperm—the male gamete cells—that can fertilise the egg (ovum). Sperm, the smallest human cells, are stored in the testicles. The testicles maintain a necessary environment for sperm survival and formation. However, sperm cells rely on semen, a fluid made of secretions from the prostate gland, seminal vesicles, and testes.

Sperm Health, Yoga, and Infertility

Sperm health is typically measured through three parameters: Quality, quantity, and motility. Unfortunately, what did not occur in the past million years is happening within a century—contemporary humans have historically the lowest sperm count and sperm quality. The reasons behind this crisis are multifaceted, including smoking, alcohol, parental alcoholism, lifestyle choices, and the presence of microplastics and pesticides in our diet (Sengupta et al., 2013; Ramlau-Hansen et al., 2007). Yoga can help address many of these issues by encouraging individuals to adopt a healthier lifestyle, reduce stress, and eliminate poor habits. It is common for people who practise yoga to embrace a healthier lifestyle. This is supported by a study concluding that yoga can improve sperm count and motility (Sengupta et al., 2013).

Female Reproductive System

With polycystic ovary syndrome and polycystic ovarian disease (PCOS/PCOD) on the rise among women, more women are adopting yoga as a potential solution. The female reproductive system is responsible for female characteristics, hormone production, ovum production, gestating and nurturing a baby. The ovaries produce ova (eggs) and hormones. The ovaries connect to the uterus through hollow muscular tubes called the fallopian tubes. The uterus is where a fertilised egg—formed by the mating of an ovum and a sperm—is implanted. The fertilised egg remains in the uterus for about 40 weeks, and from the onset of delivery, mammary glands in the breasts produce milk. The sperm cells enter through the vagina, extending from the female external genitalia to the cervix, which is responsible for childbirth and the release of menstrual fluid.

PCOS/PCOD, Yoga, and Infertility

When a pregnancy does not occur, the lining of the uterus—the endometrium—sheds and is expelled through the vagina, a process known as menstruation. Almost all women experience this once in a cycle of 22 to 31 days. However, irregular periods are gradually becoming more common, mostly due to PCOS/PCOD. PCOS/PCOD, a leading cause of infertility, is associated with hormonal imbalance, sedentary lifestyle, and stress. As observed in multiple studies, yoga is known to mitigate these factors. A systematic review has also concluded that yoga has positive effects on women suffering from PCOS/PCOD (Thakur et al., 2021). Consequently, many affected women adopt yoga as a therapeutic practice. However, as seen in males, the causes of infertility in females are also multifaceted, with poor lifestyle choices at the core. Practising yoga is recommended for infertile women because it reduces anxiety and depression. Ultimately, this improves their quality of life, contributing to a better pregnancy rate (Ha and Ban, 2021).

Every system in the body is connected with others through several feedback loops. Imbalances have cascading effects, often leading to acute or chronic conditions. Learning these systems positions us well to rectify the possible causes along with personalised yogic interventions. Through this chapter, we explored the yogic physiology and potency of yoga backed by credible research on every organ system. Moreover, these lessons also fortify our understanding of a balanced, healthy state and how yoga helps achieve it.

8

Core Concepts in Biomechanics

Biomechanics is the branch of science that deals with the mechanical aspects of motion, force, and the physical attributes of living organisms. It studies the mechanical forces acting on bones, joints, connective tissues, and other structures. Biomechanics is a sub-branch of kinesiology, which studies human movement through physiological, psychological, physical, and mental attributes.

I have seen several gym-goers with down-rotated shoulders, while they may see it as a sign of growth, I see it as a muscle imbalance. This raises the concern that awareness is scarce among coaches and individuals, or they lack proper guidance. Likewise, if unchecked, yoga practitioners are likely to develop such misalignments in their musculoskeletal structures, too. Therefore, learning biomechanics is vital for injury prevention, proper alignment, and right muscle activation, in yoga and otherwise. While injuries are uncommon in yogic practices, precautions are necessary, especially if you already have a condition or have been practising it for a long time.

Base of Support (BoS)

The base of support refers to the area of contact between the body and a supporting surface. In a typical yoga class, the legs form the base of support when they contact the mat. A wall support is also considered a base of support. A larger base of support contributes to better stability.

How do you find the base of support?

It is the total area between all points of contact that the body makes with a supporting surface (usually a yoga mat or wall).

Centre of Mass

The centre of mass of a body is the point where its entire mass acts as if it is concentrated.

Centre of Gravity

The centre of gravity of a body is the point at which all its weight acts as if it is concentrated. It is where the gravitational force appears to be concentrated. Keeping the centre of gravity within the base of support contributes to better stability. In yoga, the aim is to keep the centre of gravity aligned with the base of support. Engaging the core muscles also helps stabilise the centre of gravity.

Muscle Activation and Recruitment

Muscle activation is the process where a muscle is stimulated to generate force, initiating muscle contraction in response to the demands of a particular activity. Whereas muscle recruitment involves the simultaneous contraction of muscles to achieve stability, balance, and control in yoga positions. It refers to the process through which the nervous system initiates well-coordinated contractions of various muscles to achieve and maintain certain motions or yoga poses.

Compensation

Compensation is the phenomenon through which weakness or tightness in a muscle leads to the recruitment of other muscles or connective tissues to sustain motion. You may have experienced this before—for instance, when pushing a door, it should be easy for our triceps muscles. However, if we need to push a car, we will have to recruit several muscles. This is because, when pushing a car, our triceps muscles may not be able to generate the required amount of force, prompting other muscles to compensate. It is important to note that during compensation, we engage muscles or connective tissues that should be performing different functions.

Muscle Imbalance

Muscle imbalance results from the compensation phenomenon. In muscle imbalance, some muscles or groups of muscles are overutilised, while others are underutilised. This imbalance can also affect connective tissues, such as ligaments, tendons, and cartilage, leading to injuries.

Neuromuscular Coordination

Neuromuscular coordination is facilitated by the close interaction of muscles, the somatic nervous system (SNS), and the CNS. It allows for the precise activation and contraction of muscles through motor neurons. Proprioceptors in muscles, tendons, and joints work with the central nervous system to achieve this.

Stretching

Stretching is the process through which a muscle or connective tissue is elongated, realigning all or most of its fibres. Stretching aids in rehabilitation and increases the range of motion. Furthermore, it helps to prevent injuries by countering the compensation phenomenon, reversing the factors that diminish muscle firing. For example, the stretching of adductor muscles in Trikonasana (Triangle Pose).

Active Stretching

Active stretching is a specific type of stretching that combines elements of stretching and contraction. In terms of contraction, active stretching incorporates eccentric and isometric contractions in two phases—in phase one, eccentric (or lengthening) contraction takes place and the muscle is elongated, in phase two, the muscle remains at its new length after being subject to elongation for some time. However, this motion is neither pure eccentric contraction nor pure isometric contraction. Nonetheless, it follows the definition of stretching, where the muscle experiences 'mechanical stress'. Due to the prevalence of this phenomenon in yoga poses, I will call it 'active stretching'. For instance, the stretching of quadriceps muscles in Utkatasana (Chair Pose).

The Stretch Reflex

When a muscle is stretched, the proprioceptors signal the body to resist excessive stretching by contracting the muscle. This phenomenon is called the stretch reflex. Primarily, it is responsible for protecting the muscles. While all forms of stretching involve some contraction, conventional stretching differs from active stretching in that the contraction takes place to protect the muscles rather than to sustain movement. By practising yoga, one can ease the stretch reflex and achieve better stretches.

Proprioception and Feedback

Proprioception is the sense through which one can assess their relative body and limb positioning. It is also called kinaesthesia or body awareness. Proprioception relies greatly on proprioceptors—specialised sensory receptors located in muscles, tendons, and joints. These receptors send feedback to the CNS, leading to neuromuscular coordination. Proprioception is often confused with the sense of balance, also known as equilibrioception. Although there is considerable overlap between proprioception and equilibrioception, they are processed through separate pathways in the brain. Thus, we should not confuse these two concepts.

Joint Loading

Joint loading is defined as the force or stress applied to a joint. This force can take various forms, including compression, tension, shear, and torsion. In yoga, this force is primarily generated by movement or body weight. It is vital to assess the various joints and their surrounding ligaments, tendons, and cartilage before attempting any asana.

Joint Stability

Joint stability is the ability of a joint to withstand joint loading. It is directly linked to the condition and placement of surrounding ligaments, tendons, and cartilage. Muscles also play a critical role in stabilising a joint. Furthermore, training our muscles helps prevent excessive movement or stress on a joint.

Joint Mobility

Joint mobility is the range of motion a joint can achieve. Ideally, a joint should allow movement throughout its maximum range of motion. Joint mobility may be compromised by poor muscle health, synovial fluid, ligaments, tendons, and cartilage.

Injury Prevention

The more stable a joint is, the less likely it is to experience an injury. Therefore, to prevent injuries during a yoga class, always pay extra attention to joint loading and stability. However, joint mobility is equally important. When our joints cannot mobilise well, compensation comes into play, making our joints vulnerable. Ideally, every synovial joint should be both stable and mobile.

Arthrokinematics Motion Rule

Most synovial joints have a convex and concave surface. Based on the motion, two laws can help stabilise or mobilise our joints.

a. **The Convex-Concave Law**

   According to the convex-concave law, when the convex surface of a joint moves over the concave surface, the glide occurs in opposite directions. Understanding this law in yoga helps to stabilise the joints and prevents injuries.

   Joints that follow the convex-concave law: Knee joint, elbow joint, and ankle joint.

   Example: Hip joints in Supta Padangusthasana (Reclining Hand-to-Big-Toe Pose).

b. **The Concave-Convex Law**

   According to the concave-convex law, when the concave surface of a joint moves over the convex surface, the glide occurs in the same direction. Understanding this law in yoga helps to mobilise the joints better and achieve a greater range of motion.

   Joints that follow the concave-convex law: Shoulder joint, hip joint, and radioulnar joints. Example: Hip joints in Uttanasana (Standing Forward Bend Pose).

Kinetic Chains of Motion

Understanding the concept of kinetic chains of motion enhances one's perspective on various poses and their variations in yoga. This knowledge compels us to make more informed decisions in reaching our goals in yoga. There are two types of kinetic chains of movements—open kinetic chain movements and closed kinetic chain movements.

a. **Open Kinetic Chain Movement**

   In open kinetic chain movements, some distal limbs do not contact any surface. Consequently, the base of support is typically less. The lack of a base of support is compensated for by greater activation of agonist and antagonist muscles. Overall, open kinetic chain movements allow a greater scope for isolated joint movements and muscle training.

   Example: Utkatasana (Chair Pose), Virabhadrasana I (Warrior I Pose), Virabhadrasana III (Warrior III Pose), etc.

b. **Closed Kinetic Chain Motion**

   In closed kinetic chain movements, most, if not all, distal limbs make contact with a surface (including the body). As a result, the base of support is typically greater. A higher degree of coordinated effort between agonist and antagonist muscles is required here. Closed kinetic chain movements are much more functional and biomechanically efficient as they resemble real-life movements.

   Examples: Phalakasana (Plank Pose), Setu bandhasana (Bridge Pose), Balasana (Child's Pose), etc.

In conclusion, no movements are identical, and no asanas are the same. For instance, although Uttanasana and Ardha Uttanasana may appear similar, they differ significantly, as we'll explore in the upcoming chapters. The effectiveness of an asana depends on the practitioner's goals. A movement can be efficient or inefficient based on the effort required and the benefits gained relative to the intended objective. Biomechanics and kinesiology are science-backed parameters used to assess movement. An informed yoga practitioner can use these principles to carefully design the right yoga flow to achieve their desired goal.

Section III

Untwining the Asanas

Have you ever wondered how these simple-looking asanas work? How do asanas integrate mobility, flexibility, strength, and agility?

Take your breath as an anchor and delve deeper into the biomechanics and kinesiology of asanas. In this segment, we will learn more than 50 asanas while infusing muscle actions, joint actions, modifications, progression, regression, prop work, and much more. Completing this segment should allow you to decode every asana possible. Imagine the power of the X-ray vision of asanas to maximise your gains.

9

Foundational Asanas: The Path to Inner Peace

In the foundational asanas, I have covered poses that are essential to yogic practices. These poses are ideal for achieving a tranquil mind. Practising these asanas brings an instant sense of gratitude and stillness. Additionally, these movements also evoke a sense of groundedness and positivity.

FOUNDATIONAL STANDING ASANAS

Imagine sitting for far too long, causing stress to the spine and surrounding tissues. You can decompress the spine and tissues by practising simple standing asanas, such as Tadasana, Samasthiti, and Namaskarasana.

Tadasana directly translates to 'Palm Tree Pose', not Mountain Pose. It involves stretching the arms upwards while balancing the body on the toes. Similarly, the Mountain Pose should be called Samasthiti or 'Equal Standing Pose', which resembles the standard anatomical position. It is a practice for cultivating an equanimous mind. Moreover, Namaskarasana is the posture where we assume the Namaskara Mudra, or Anjali Mudra (Salutation Gesture), in Samasthiti. It is mainly practised in the 1st and 12th positions of the traditional Hatha Surya Namaskar (Sun Salutation). These three asanas are collectively known as the foundational standing asanas.

Samasthiti (Equal Standing Pose)

Etymology: *Sama* means equal; *Sthiti* means standing or state of being.

Asana Category	Targeted Area	Preparatory Yogic Practices
Standing	Spine (axial extension)	
Beginner-friendly	Shoulder joints (flexion) (except Samasthiti)	
Balancing	Elbow joints (extension)	None
-	Hip joints (extension)	
-	Knee joints (extension)	

Technique:

a. Begin by assuming a normal standing position.

b. Gently, keep your legs about hip-width apart.

c. Next, firmly grip all your toes and heels down on the mat, ensuring that all your toes press into the ground. Meanwhile, also ensure an equal distribution of weight on the toes and heels of both legs.

d. Keep a micro-flexion (micro-bend) in your knees.

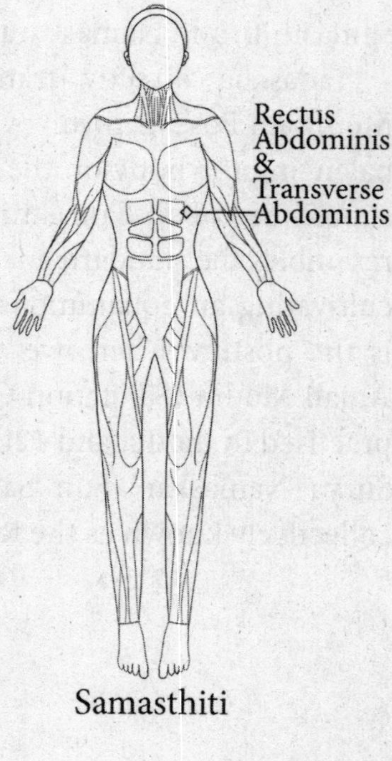

Samasthiti

e. (Inhale) Start engaging your quadriceps muscles (the front thigh muscles) to the maximum extent possible. While doing so, your kneecaps (patellae) should be pulled upwards.

f. (Exhale) Maintain a gentle posterior tilt by engaging the lower abdomen. Ensure that your spine remains almost neutral.

g. (Inhale) Now, move your shoulders up, back, and down. Retract the scapulae and allow your chest to open.

h. (Continue inhalation) Open all your fingers while pointing them down towards the ground.

i. (Exhale) Tuck your navel and chin slightly inwards.

j. (Normal breath) Maintain this position for about 10–20 breaths or relax if you experience fatigue in the muscles surrounding your shoulder blades or toes.

Namaskarasana (Salutation Pose)

Etymology: *Namaskara* means salutation or greeting; *Asana* means pose or posture.

Technique:

a. Start by assuming Samasthiti (Equal Standing Pose).

b. From here, gently join your palms together in Namaskar or Anjali Mudra (Salutation Gesture).

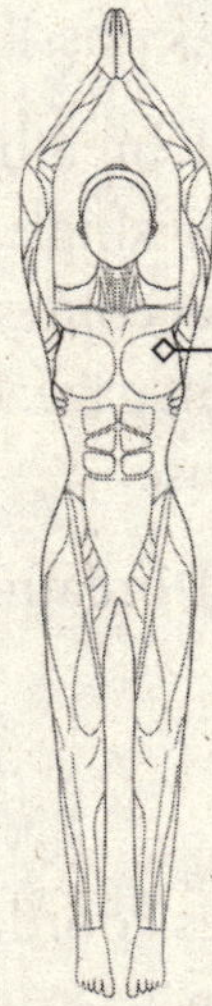

Namaskarasana

Tadasana (Palm Tree Pose)

Etymology: *Tada* translates to mountain; *Asana* means pose or posture.

Technique:

a. Begin by assuming Samasthiti.

b. From here, lift your shoulders forward and interlace your fingers.

c. (Inhale) Lift your shoulders all the way up while stretching your arms towards the sky or ceiling. In the process, ensure you do not hunch or curve your back.

d. (Continue inhalatison) When you feel ready, lift your heels as high as possible.

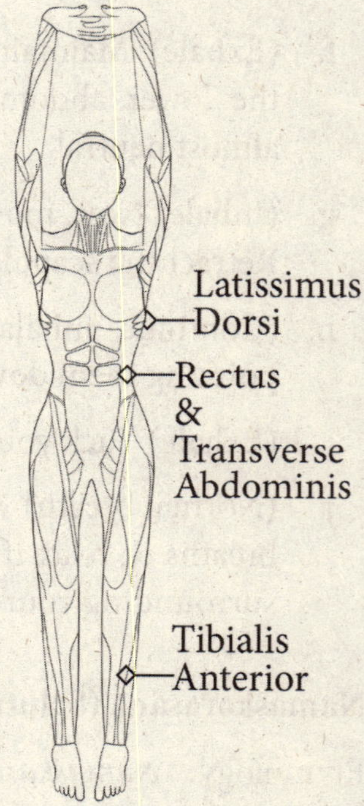

Tadasana

e. (Normal breath) If possible, choose a single non-moving point that comes directly into your line of sight; maintain a constant gaze. Doing so will improve focus and stability in the pose.

f. (Normal breath) Assume this posture for about 5–15 breaths.

Benefits

- Improves coordination between the two hemispheres of the brain

- Improves groundedness of the feet
- Improves digestion
- Heightens awareness level
- Stretches the entire body
- Releases pressure from various joints
- Improves the weight perception of our body
- Improves mindfulness
- Maintains the natural arch of the feet

Common Mistakes to Avoid

- Externally rotating the legs
- Hunching or arching the back
- Protruding the chin
- Putting unequal weight on both legs
- Lifting the inner or outer side of the foot

Biomechanics

The axial extension of the spine is usually considered good practice while assuming Tadasana, Samasthiti, or Namaskarasana. Tucking the chin slightly inwards helps to keep the cervical spine neutral.

The rhomboid and trapezius muscles help draw the shoulder blades (scapulae) towards the midline of the body, which helps to open the chest area. To maintain a neutral spine, the erector spinae and transversospinalis muscles work in tandem with the abdominal muscles (core muscles).

The rotator cuff muscles ensure the safety and stability of the glenohumeral joint (shoulder joint), which is more unstable compared to most other synovial joints. While assuming Palm Tree Pose, if you experience tightness in the arms or have a frozen shoulder, it may be advisable to practise it with Namaskar Mudra in front. It is so because raising the arms overhead can place the shoulder articular capsules—important for smooth movement—between the acromion process and the humerus, causing discomfort.

The calf muscles, primarily the soleus and gastrocnemius, play their part in preventing us from falling forward. Hence, they actively participate in these asanas. Strong calf muscles ensure better stability.

Additionally, the gluteal muscles also stabilise movement by keeping the body upright. In fact, humans have larger gluteal muscles than other animals because we learnt to walk upright. These same muscles show their strength in these asanas as well.

Modifications

Samasthiti can also be practised with both legs joined together. This position helps to keep the centre of gravity close to the feet.

FOUNDATIONAL DHYANATMAK ASANA (MEDITATIVE POSTURES)

Dhyanatmak asanas (meditative postures) have been depicted in the second chapter (Sadhana Pada) of the Patanjali Yoga Sutra, through the following Sutra:

Sthira Sukham Asanam [2.46]

It translates to, a position where one feels stability and comfort is an asana. Here, Maharshi Patanjali ji is primarily talking about the meditative asanas.

Meditative postures include Sukhasana (Easy Pose), Ardha Padmasana (Half Lotus Pose), Swastikasana (Auspicious Pose),

Siddhasana (Accomplished Pose), Padmasana (Lotus Pose), Vajrasana (Thunderbolt Pose), and Virasana (Hero Pose). Out of these, Sukhasana and Ardha Padmasana (Half Lotus Pose) are the easiest. Mostly because they are asymmetrical, unlike other meditative asanas. Yet, they are not depicted in the most ancient yogic scriptures. Whereas Padmasana, Swastikasana, and Siddhasana have been mentioned in various ancient yogic scriptures with great emphasis. Padmasana is named after the lotus, a sacred flower, and a symbol of prosperity and wisdom. Similarly, Swastikasana is named after the auspicious symbol of *Swastika*. Although it has been revered among Eastern cultures for more than 2–3 millenniums, the widespread misinformation around Swastika is tremendous. Additionally, Siddhasana bestows positivity and wisdom to whoever practices it.

Asana Category	Targeted Area	Preparatory Yogic Practices
Meditative	Spine (axial extension)	Dandasana (Staff Pose)
Sitting	Shoulder joints (flexion)	Sukhasana (Easy Pose)
Cross-legged	Hip joint (external rotation) (flexion) (abduction)	Ardha Padmasana
Beginner-friendly	Knee joints (flexion)	-
-	Ankle joints (plantar flexion) (eversion)	-

Dandasana (Staff Pose)

Etymology: *Danda* means staff or stick; *Asana* means posture.

Technique:

a. Sit on the yoga mat and extend your legs in front of you.
b. Keep your arms resting at your sides, with your elbows slightly flexed and palms resting on the ground.
c. Create a slight anterior tilt to maintain an erect spine.
d. Tuck your toes in slightly.

Sukhasana (Easy Pose)

Etymology: *Sukha* means happiness or ease; *Asana* translates to pose.

Technique:

a. From Dandasana, bend your knees in an easy cross-legged position.
b. First, externally rotate and flex your right knee, placing it under your left thigh.
c. Similarly, externally rotate and flex the left knee, placing it under your right thigh. This will cross your legs.

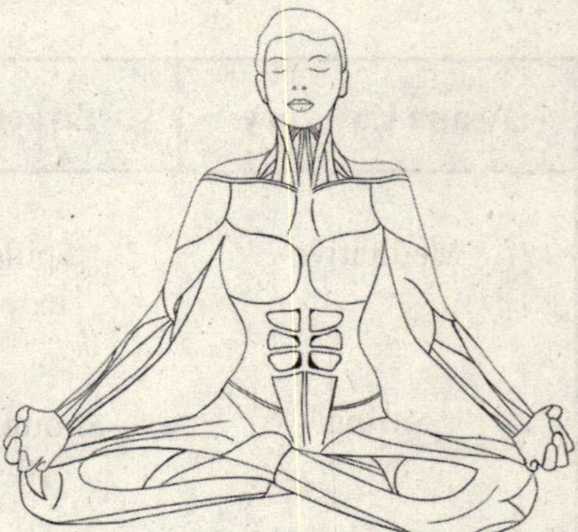
Sukhasana

Ardha Padmasana (Half Lotus Pose)

Etymology: *Ardha* means half; *Padma* means lotus; *Asana* means posture or seat.

Technique:

a. From Dandasana, externally rotate and flex your right knee, placing it on the top of your left thigh.

b. Externally rotate and flex your left knee, placing it under your right thigh. This will not cross your legs.

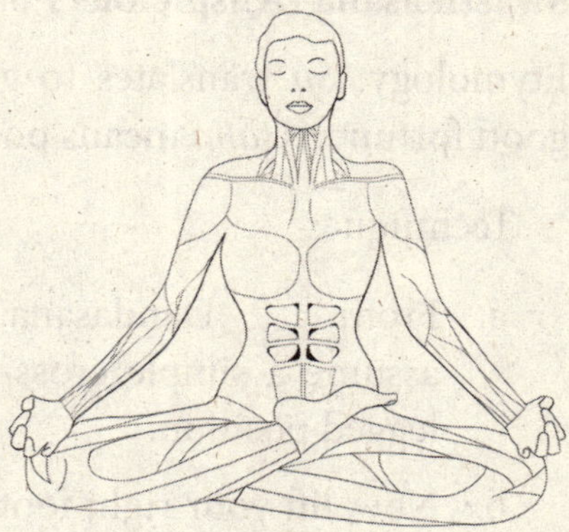

Ardha Padmasana

Siddhasana (Accomplished Pose)

Etymology: *Siddha* means accomplished or perfected; *Asana* translates to posture or seat.

Technique:

a. From Dandasana, externally rotate and flex your left knee, placing the left heel close to your pelvis.

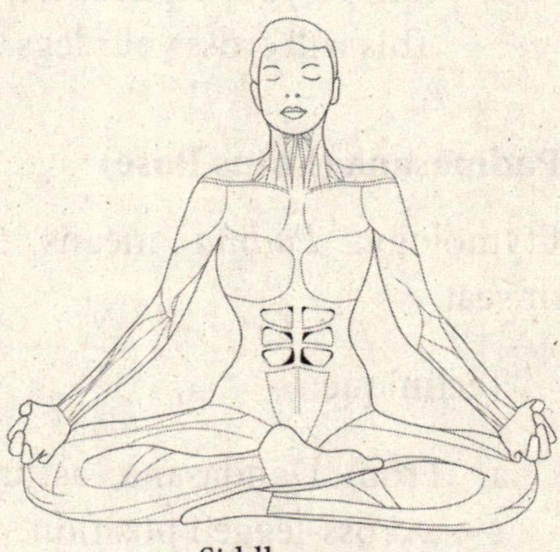

Siddhasana

b. Similarly, externally rotate and flex your right knee, placing your right heel over the left one. This will not cross your legs.

Swastikasana (Auspicious Pose)

Etymology: *Su* translates to good; *asti* means well-being or good fortune; *Asana* means posture or seat.

Technique:

a. From Dandasana, assume a simple cross-legged position.

b. Now, lift your right foot and place it under the fold of your left knee.

c. Next, take your left knee and place it under the fold of your right knee. This will cross your legs.

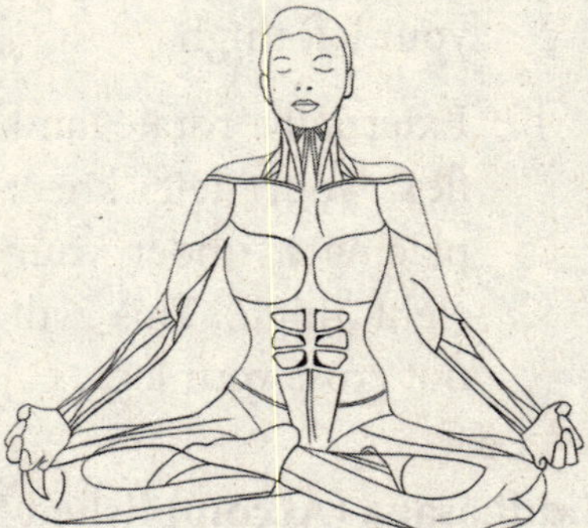

Swastikasana

Padmasana (Lotus Pose)

Etymology: *Padma* means lotus; *Asana* means posture or seat.

Technique:

a. From Dandasana, assume a cross-legged position.

b. Externally rotate and flex your left knee, placing it on top of your right thigh.

c. Likewise, externally rotate and flex your right knee, placing it on top of your left thigh. This will cross your legs.

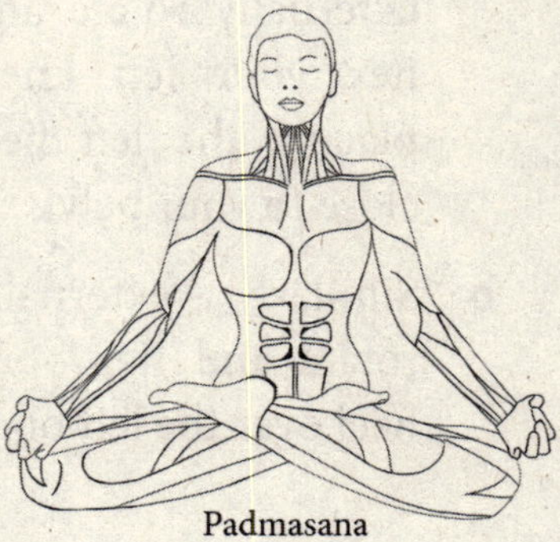

Padmasana

d. After assuming the meditative posture, take deep breaths and keep your spine long, placing your hands comfortably on your knees with the Hasta Mudra (hand gesture/lock) of your choice.

Beginners should hold each Asana for 5 to 15 minutes during yoga practice.

Benefits

- Settles the mind
- Benefits gut health
- Balances the autonomic system response
- Relieves stress, anxiety, and depression
- Boosts mood
- Helps meditate
- Stretches hip muscles
- Helps in practising pranayama
- Develops body and breath connection
- Improves the respiratory system
- Enhances self-awareness and somatosensory perception

Common Mistakes to Avoid

- Not mobilising your hip joints
- Flexing the spine
- Protruding the neck forward
- Sitting on an uneven surface
- Elevating the shoulders
- Assuming any asana for far too long

Biomechanics

Due to prolonged sitting, several back muscles tend to tense, and downward-rotated shoulders become prominent. To prevent this, aim for strong back and abdominal muscles. Furthermore, keep your spine neutral and your shoulder blades up and not down.

Ideally, to maintain an erect spine, the erector spinae muscle group, along with the transversospinalis muscle group, should contract to keep the spine extended. Moreover, the abdominal muscles also contribute to trunk stability.

People often experience difficulty while practising meditative postures due to two main reasons: anatomical variations in the hip, knee, and ankle joint structures and tightness in the medial rotators of the hip, especially the gluteus medius, gluteus minimus, and tensor fascia latae. The goal is to achieve most hip joint rotation from the hip joint itself. Thus, hip stretches before practice are advised. In this context, the sartorius muscles assist with external rotation at the hips and flexion at the knees, while the deep hip external rotators aid in the external rotation of the hip. However, tight hamstrings can pose certain challenges, especially for the knee joint.

Lastly, dorsiflexion of the foot is facilitated by the soleus muscles, whereas supination in the ankle joints causes the fibularis muscles to stretch.

Modifications

- While sitting, ensure an anterior tilt for an erect spine as it is less susceptible to injury, especially of spinal origin. To achieve this, place the sit bones (ischial tuberosity) slightly higher than the knees. You can use yoga props like yoga blocks, yoga blankets, and others.

Vajrasana (Thunderbolt Pose) and Virasana (Hero Pose)

If easy digestion is the one thing you ask for, look no further than Vajrasana and Virasana. The popularity of these asanas is evident in numerous traditions across the world. In fact, in Eastern traditions, including Japanese and Indian cultures, people prefer to eat in these positions. Additionally, in ancient yogic texts, Vajrasana is the only asana that can also be

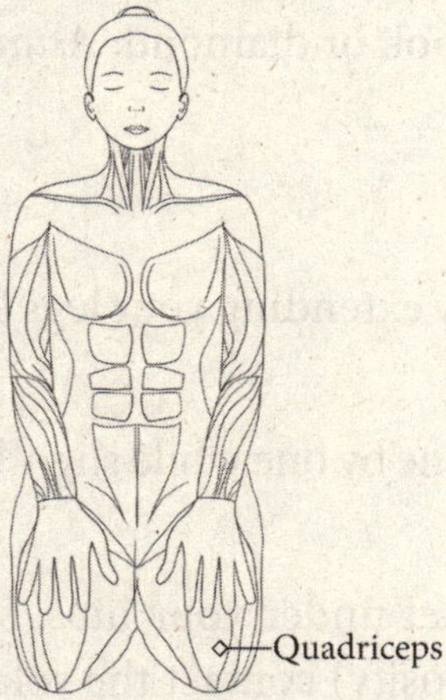

Vajrasana

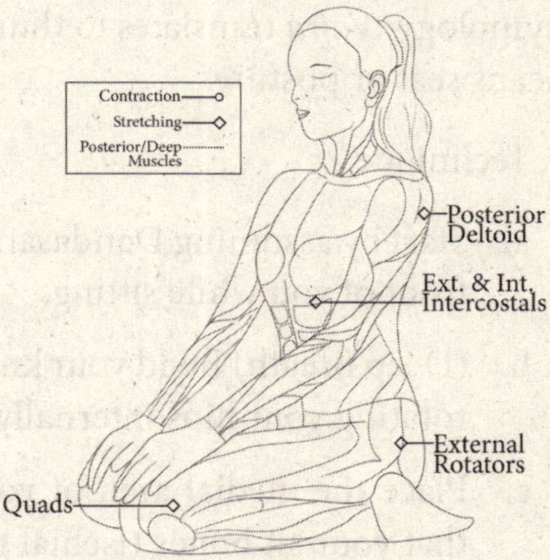

Virasana

Asana Category	Targeted Area	Preparatory Yogic Practices
Meditative	Spine (axial extension)	Dandasana (Staff Pose)
Sitting	Shoulder joints (flexion)	Sukshma Vyayama (Pre-practices)
Beginner-friendly	Hip joints (internal rotation) (flexion) (adduction)	
	Knee joints (flexion)	
	Ankle joints (plantar flexion) (iversion)	

practised after meals to improve digestion. These meditative postures may seem similar but are unique in their own way. Vajrasana, for instance, is comparatively easy to perform—it keeps the spine in better and much more neutral alignment, while Virasana focuses more on stretching our deep pelvic and quadriceps muscles and can be difficult for many individuals.

Vajrasana (Thunderbolt Pose)

Etymology: *Vajra* translates to thunderbolt or diamond; *Asana* means seat or posture.

Technique:

a. Start by assuming Dandasanxa by extending your legs in front of you while sitting.

b. (Deep Breath) Bend your knees one by one while slightly rotating your hips internally.

c. Place the medial arch of your feet under your hips, so that your sit bones (ischial tuberosity) contact the soles of your feet. Your big toes (preferably the right big toe over the left) should touch.

Virasana (Hero Pose)

Etymology: *Vira* means hero or warrior; *Asana* means posture.

Technique:

a. Take a deep breath and bend your knees one by one while slightly rotating your hips internally.

b. Make sure to place the arches of your feet alongside your hips so that your sit bones touch the floor.

c. After assuming the pose, take a deep breath and keep your spine long and place your hands comfortably on your knees or assume the Hasta Mudra (hand gesture/ lock) of your choice.

d. Stay in this position for as long as you feel comfortable, a maximum of 5 to 10 minutes.

Benefits

- Improves digestion
- Improves the reproductive system response
- Improves tidal volume (lung capacity)
- Increases concentration
- Brings a sense of comfort
- Improves Prana Shakti
- Deepens the state of meditation
- Mobilises the ankle joints
- Helps alleviate asthma and hypertension
- Boosts mindfulness

Common Mistakes to Avoid

- Straining your ankle, knee, and hip joints
- Not mobilising your ankle, knee, and hip joints correctly

Biomechanics

While assuming Vajrasana, our pelvis naturally takes a neutral position. Hence, we usually have an elongated (axial extension) spine. Conversely, in Virasana, our pelvis may tilt posteriorly. Thus, we often observe a rounded back.

Depression of shoulders and retraction of scapula blades can be a good idea that can help open your chest muscles.

In both asanas, sometimes, a few individuals struggle because of their limited ankle joint mobility. In such cases, I recommend mobilising the ankles properly and giving them time to adapt. However, for some, their ankles are anatomically designed to not allow full plantar flexion. If you experience something like this, you can switch to more comfortable meditative postures, such as Sukhasana (Easy Pose).

If you experience tightness in the front thigh, it could be due to tight quadriceps or gluteal muscles.

For individuals with low-back pain, internal rotation of the hip joints can be helpful. This occurs because tight external rotators often cause pelvic instability, resulting in pain.

Modifications

- **Regression:** Those who experience mild discomfort in the knees can also use a folded yoga blanket and sandwich it between their calf muscles and thighs. This will help restrict the motion, alleviating discomfort.
- **Prop Work:** In Virasana, to maintain an upright spine, it is better to place a yoga prop, such as a yoga block, yoga bolster, or yoga blanket under your hips. Doing so will help you maintain the anterior pelvic tilt, resulting in an upright spine. Furthermore, the same practice also works for people who experience mild knee discomfort.

Baddha Konasana (Bound Angle Pose)

Etymology: *Baddha* means bound; *Kona* translates to angle; *Asana* means posture.

Baddha Konasana, also known as the Bound Angle Pose, may seem trivial but can prevent the 'dead butt syndrome' that can arise from persistent sitting. It causes the tightening of hip muscles and may later interfere with the spine. If your job requires you to sit for long hours, it is essential to add Baddha Konasana to your everyday life. It is also easy to do and among the popular beginner-friendly asanas. The dynamic version of this asana is also sometimes referred to as the Titliasana (Butterfly Pose).

In this asana, your tibialis anterior and adductors are actively stretched.

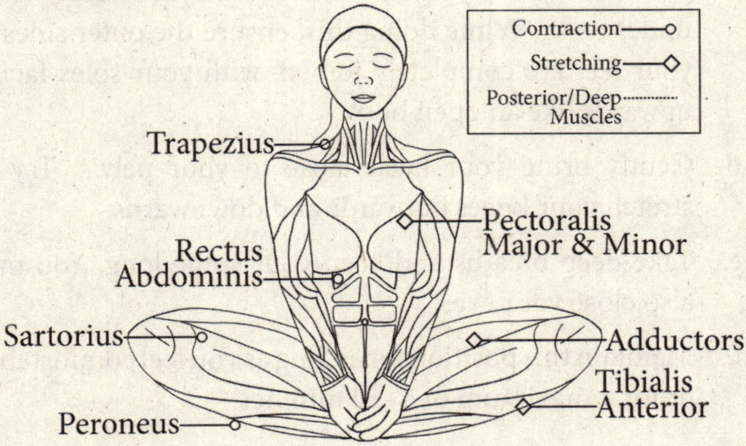

Baddhakonasana

Asana Category	Targeted Area	Preparatory Yogic Practices
Meditative	Spine (axial extension)	Sukhasana (Easy Pose)
Sitting	Pelvis (anterior pelvic tilt)	Agnistambhasana (Fire Log Pose)
Beginner-friendly	Hip joint (external rotation)	
	Hip joint (flexion)	
	Hip joint (abduction)	
	Knee joints (flexion)	

Technique:

a. Assume Dandasana (Staff Pose) and extend your legs while sitting on the yoga mat. Tilt your pelvis anteriorly by moving your hips back.

b. Bring your feet together and bend your knees, allowing your legs to move outward—this involves abduction and external rotation of the hip joints.

c. Interlace your fingers and hold your feet from underneath. While doing this, ensure the outer sides of your feet are completely joined, with your soles facing upwards like an open book.

d. Gently bring your heels close to your pelvis. Try to stretch your knees outwards and downwards.

e. Take deep breaths and keep your spine long. You may also close your eyes.

f. Maintain this position for as long as you feel comfortable, or for a maximum of 5–10 minutes.

Benefits

- Stretches groin muscles
- Enhances pelvic floor muscle function
- Improves digestive health
- Alleviates stress perception
- Prepares for a longer meditative session
- Improves reproductive functions
- Stretches the inner thigh muscles (adductors).
- Helps prevent the dead butt syndrome
- Enhances the mobility of the hip joints
- Calms the mind

Common Mistakes to Avoid

- Not mobilising your hip joints

- Flexing the spine
- Jutting the neck forward
- Sitting on an uneven surface
- Elevating the shoulders

Biomechanics

Ideally, your knees should touch the floor, pointing forward. If your knees are lifted off in this asana, it could mean you have tight hip muscles. However, bio-individuality could be the reason and not tight hip muscles. This is completely normal.

Baddha Konasana depends on abdominal muscles for the descent of the legs against gravity as iliopsoas muscles cannot control it effectively. This may cause excessive spinal extension, which needs to be regulated.

Press your feet beneath to activate fibularis muscles.

A minimal stretch while assuming this asana could symbolise hypermobility (possibly due to loose ligaments), and in that case, it is better to focus on strengthening asanas.

Depression of the shoulders and retraction of scapula blades can be a good idea and will help stretch your chest muscles.

The gluteal and hip external rotator muscles contract to form abduction and external rotation of the hips. Meanwhile, the hips' internal rotators stabilise the movement. This allows the adductor muscles to stretch.

To stabilise the spine, the erector spinae muscle group works with the transversospinalis, quadratus lumborum, and abdominal (core) muscles.

Modifications

- In case your knees are lifted off and causing you discomfort, you can use yoga props such as blocks, bolsters, and blankets underneath your knees.

- To maintain an anterior tilt while sitting, it's important to ensure that you have an upright spine that is less prone to injury, especially of spinal origin. To achieve this, it is helpful to position the sit bones slightly higher than the feet. Yoga props such as yoga blocks and blankets can be used to assist with this.

Balasana (Child's Pose)

Etymology: *Bal* translates to child; *Asana* means pose or posture

We all seek a refreshing and rejuvenating asana after a long day at work. Balasana, also known as the Child's Pose, is among the restorative asanas that help rest the body after an exhausting day. It stretches our key muscles like the back, hips, and front thigh muscles—which are among the most overworked muscles. Furthermore, the Child's Pose is also among the postures that aid in digestion and bring serenity to the mind.

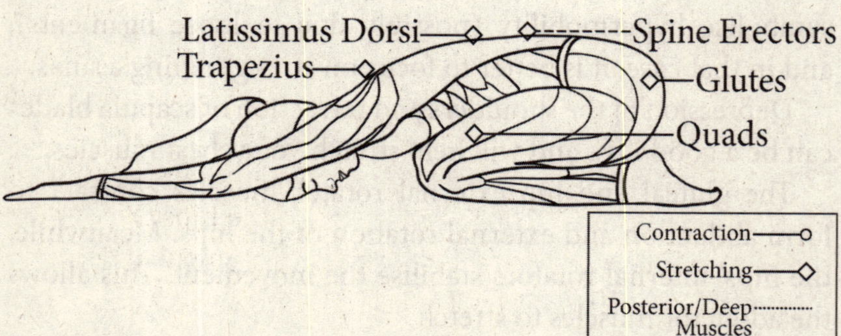

Balasana

Technique:

a. Begin by assuming Dandasana.

b. One by one, flex your knees and place your feet under your hips. Do this so that you sit on the heels and the medial side of your feet. Keep your spine upright.

c. Exhale and move your hips slightly back. Place your palms in front of your knees and slide them forward while bending forward (trunk flexion).

d. Gently, if your body allows, lower your forehead to the mat. Meanwhile, ensure your hips remain grounded.

e. Take deep breaths and allow gravity to hold your body rather than holding yourself up. Surrender completely to the ground. Hold the pose for 10–20 breaths, staying mindful of the stretches.

f. Follow the instructions in reverse to come out of the pose.

Asana Category	Targeted Area	Preparatory Yogic Practices
Beginner-friendly	Spine (flexion)	Vajrasana (Thunderbolt Pose)
Sitting	Shoulder joints (flexion)	Virasana (Hero Pose)
Forward bend	Elbow joints (flexion)	-
Inversion/upside down	Hip joints (flexion)	
	Knee joints (flexion)	
	Ankle joints (plantar flexion)	

Benefits

- Helps restore the PNS dominance
- Aids improving digestion
- Relaxes the spine and surrounding tissues
- Stretches muscles, including the back, hips, front thighs, and shin muscles

- Relaxes muscles that tend to tighten, especially due to a sedentary lifestyle
- Calms both the mind and body
- Brings a sense of humility
- Helps counter work-related fatigue, stress, and anxiety

Common Mistakes to Avoid

- Lifting your hips off the heels
- Forcing your neck down
- Discomfort in your neck and head

Biomechanics

Child's Pose is primarily a passive stretch and is based on a closed kinetic chain (CKC) motion. It is an excellent example of surrendering the body to Mother Earth (gravity), with the entire movement being gravity-assisted.

Practitioners with less mobile ankles and weak toe extensors should mobilise their ankles through Sukshma Vyayama before assuming the pose.

It stretches key muscles, including the erector spinae, transversospinalis, latissimus dorsi, trapezius, quadriceps, tibialis anterior, and the gluteal muscles (maximus, medius, and minimus).

If you experience difficulty reaching your trunk forward to the mat, it is highly likely that you need to work on your hip muscles. For this, practise hip-opening asanas such as Utthan Pristhasana (Lizard Pose).

Often, tightness in the back muscles (QL and spinal muscles) can limit flexion, leading to a restricted forward bend in this asana.

Cramps in and around the foot are often caused by weak posterior intrinsic muscles of the foot (extensor digitorum brevis and extensor hallucis brevis). To overcome this, try activating the toes before practising.

Lastly, if your breathing feels restricted, open your knees slightly or ease into a more regressed version of the pose.

Modifications

- **Variation I:** If you find it difficult to place your head on the mat or if doing so causes your hips to lift off the ground, form fists with your hands, stack them on top of each other, and place your head on the uppermost fist. Alternatively, you can place a yoga block or bolster in front of you.
- **Variation II:** You can relax your arms by your sides, with your head turned to either side.
- **Regression:** If the stretch feels too intense, you can limit the forward bending and stop halfway, using your arms to support your body.
- **Progression:** You can widen your knees to allow more space for your trunk to rest. This creates an additional stretch while providing more room for your belly (diaphragm) to breathe.
- **Prop Work:** If you experience cramps in your soles (usually caused by toe extensors) or discomfort in your ankles, you can roll a towel or yoga blanket under your ankles.
- **Yin Yoga:** You can place a yoga bolster in front of you to support your head and help you relax.

10
Bowing to Stillness: Forward-Bending Asanas for Mind and Body

Forward-bending poses promote introspection by focusing on the natural curve of the spine. These poses are essential in yoga and understanding their benefits and biomechanics can enhance our practice.

Ardha Uttanasana (Standing Half Forward Bend Pose)

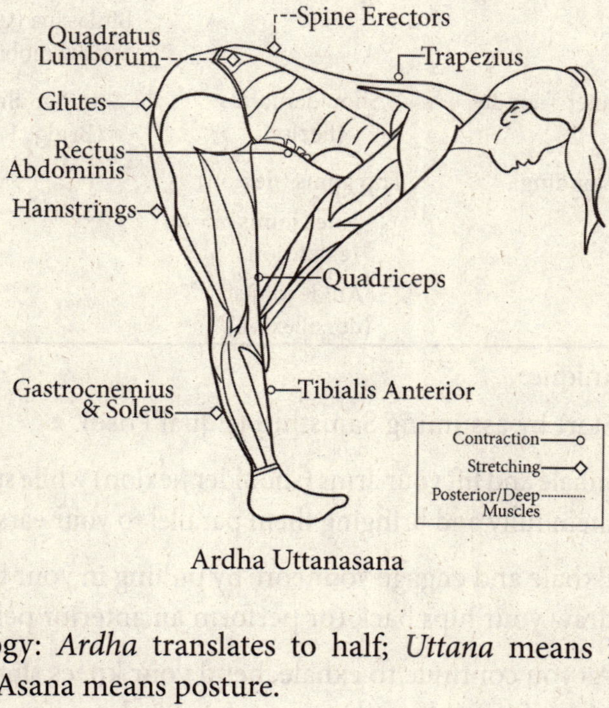

Ardha Uttanasana

Etymology: *Ardha* translates to half; *Uttana* means intense stretch; Asana means posture.

Ardha Uttanasana can improve our functional fitness (Gothe and Edward 2016) by stretching and strengthening. People often believe that Ardha Uttanasana and Uttanasana function identically as both are hamstring stretches. However, there are notable differences, which we will discuss later in this chapter.

In this asana, the hamstrings, glutes (maximus, medius, and minimus), erector spinae, transversospinalis, quadratus lumborum, gastrocnemius, and soleus are stretched, with some experiencing active engagement, depending on the practitioner's focus and alignment.

Asana Category	Targeted Area	Preparatory Yogic Practices
Forward-bending	Spine (flexion)	Marjaryasana and Bitilasana (Cat and Cow mobility)
Beginner-friendly	Shoulder joints (flexion)	Setu Bandhasana (Bridge Pose)
Standing	Hip joints (flexion) Knee joints (extension) Ankle joints (dorsiflexion)	

Technique:

a. Start by assuming Samsthiti (Equal Pose).

b. Inhale and lift your arms (shoulder flexion) while stretching them fully and bringing them parallel to your ears.

c. Exhale and engage your core by pulling in your belly and draw your hips back (or perform an anterior pelvic tilt).

d. As you continue to exhale, bend your knees slightly and hinge forward until you reach a 90-degree angle, or as far as you can without rounding your spine.

e. Breathe normally and keep your arms and neck (cervical spine) aligned with the rest of your spine. Gently rest your arms on your thighs.

f. Continue to lengthen your spine by drawing your hips further back and moving your neck slightly forward.

g. Hold this asana for 5 to 10 breaths.

h. Reverse the steps to come out of the pose.

Benefits

- Strengthens the posterior chain of muscles, including the spine erector muscles, glutes, hamstrings, and calf muscles
- Stretches the hamstring, calf, and Hip muscles
- Improves overall body posture
- Enhances blood circulation through diffusion
- Furthers the suppleness of the spine and hips
- Activates rotator cuff muscles
- Strengthens neck muscles

Common Mistakes to Avoid

- Hunching your back—it can result in injuries
- Looking forward, as it puts strain on neck muscles
- Hyperextending your knees

Biomechanics

Ardha Uttanasana is among the asanas where you can feel the difference between a closed kinetic chain motion and an open kinetic chain motion. The major difference between Ardha Uttanasana and Uttanasana is that on a scale of 10—Ardha Uttanasana is fighting 9/10 against gravity, whereas Uttanasana is fighting 3/10 against gravity. Here, we are shifting our centre of gravity forward, and to counteract this, our body engages various muscles.

Unlike Uttanasana, Ardha Uttanasana involves active hamstring stretch where it (especially, the biceps femoris) lengthens while resisting the motion against gravity. Here, activation of the iliopsoas muscle is almost irrelevant. Thus, it mostly remains passive. However, to maintain an extended knee, the quadriceps muscles activate. Meanwhile, the tibialis anterior muscles work in conjunction with the opposing soleus and gastrocnemius muscles to ensure dorsiflexion of the ankle joints, preventing a forward fall.

In Ardha Uttanasana, the gluteal muscles are also stretched while contracting.

In Uttanasana, the spine erector muscles contract while lengthening instead of passively stretching. This is to resist the natural gravitational pull. The back muscles work as a stabiliser as gravity initiates the movement, and the transverse abdominis muscles also work in tandem with the back muscles. Hence, in Ardha Uttanasana, the posterior (back) chain of muscles is contracted while lengthening and the anterior chain of muscles remains relatively relaxed.

Make sure to maintain an anterior pelvic tilt to support the weight bearing. Focus on keeping your spine neutral rather than extending your knees. If your spine starts to round, don't hesitate to bend your knees. Your knees should be slightly bent to stretch the hamstrings, otherwise, only the sciatic nerve will stretch.

Modifications

- **Variation I:** The Ardha Uttanasana can also be performed by placing your hands parallel to the floor. This variation is especially recommended for practitioners who wish to progress into the stretches.

- **Variation II:** This asana can also be practised by keeping your upper limbs parallel to the spine and adjacent to the body (often called airplane arms). This variation is recommended for practitioners who have been practising yoga for some time.
- **Variation III:** Ardha Uttanasana can also be performed while placing your arms completely on the mat. However, according to me, it is only meant for advanced practitioners with an extensively mobile pelvic area and surrounding tissues.
- **Regression:** If you find this asana to be intense, you can regress by bending your knees slightly.
- **Progression:** If you have been practising yoga for some time and wish to progress into the asana, bring your arms forward and shift your body weight (centre of gravity) towards your toes.
- **Wall Support:** You can also practise this asana with the support of a wall.
- **Prop Work:** You can add a yoga block between your thighs to engage your hip internal rotators, as it helps redirect motion only to the hip flexion.

Uttanasana (Standing Forward Bend)

Etymology: Uttan means intense stretch; asana translates to pose.

Uttanasana stretches the hamstrings, but should we really be stretching them? Stretching a tight hamstring without understanding the underlying cause of its tightness can be misguided. Often, the hamstrings tighten as a protective response when the spine is under unprovoked strain, such as from slouching or swayback (lordosis), to preventlow back pain. Therefore, it's advisable to first mobilise the lower spine and surrounding muscles before attempting Uttanasana.

Active Stretch: Gluteal (maximus, medius, and minimus), soleus, gastrocnemius, and tibialis posterior.

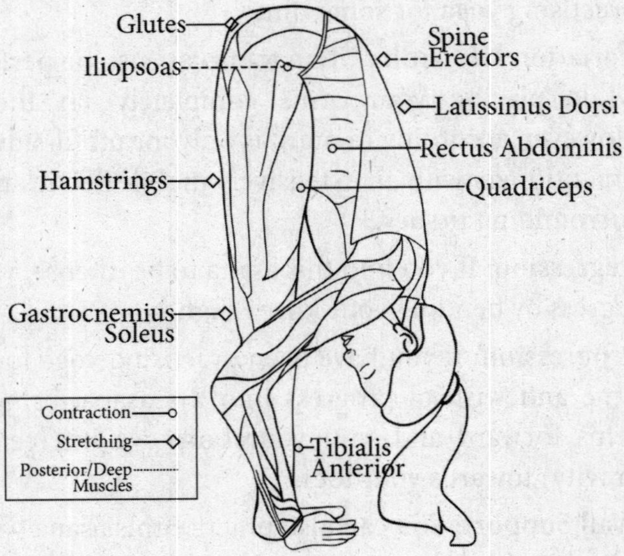

Uttanasana

Asana Category	Targeted Area	Preparatory Yogic Practices
Beginner-friendly	Spine (flexion)	Ardha Uttanasana (Halfway Standing Forward Bend Pose)
Forward bend	Shoulder joints (flexion)	Dandasana (Staff Pose)
Hamstring stretch	Elbow joints (extension)	Janusirsasana (Head-To-Knee Pose)
Standing	Pelvis (posterior pelvic tilt)	
	Hip joints (flexion)	
	Knee joints (extension)	

Technique:

a. Begin with Tadasana or Samsthiti (Equal Standing).
b. Evenly distribute your body weight on both your legs and ensure a symmetrical position.
c. Inhale and lift your arms over your head—by flexing your shoulder. Try to lengthen your spine as much as you can. Make a hook with your first two fingers by curling them in your hands.
d. Exhale and move your tailbone outwards (anterior pelvic tilt) and gradually bend forward.
e. Maintain the anterior tilt to about 90 degrees of trunk fold (flexion) and avoid rounding your back as much as possible.
f. Continue exhaling beyond 90 degrees of trunk fold (flexion) and allow your spine to gradually round.
g. Now, from the hook of your index and middle fingers catch your big toes (only if your body allows you).
h. Breathe normally, and hold this position for 10 to 20 seconds or as per your capacity. Gently return to the Tadasana. Repeat it 3 to 5 times

Benefits

- Improves flexibility of the spine
- Furthers blood circulation to the spinal discs
- Improves strength and functions of the spinal ligaments
- Helps prevent osteoporosis by strengthening the bones and muscles
- Counterbalances backbends
- Assist with retrospection

Common Mistakes to Avoid

- Steep forward bends, especially from your lower back (L4-L5 and L5-S1)
- Forcing the head to the knees
- Looking towards the toes
- Hyperextending the knee
- Externally rotating (moving outwards) your legs

Biomechanics

The degree of pelvic tilt is crucial in Uttanasana. Therefore, it is important to assess the degree of pelvic tilt beforehand. You can practise Marjaryasana and Bitilasana (cat and cow stretches).

When you catch your big toes with your index and middle fingers, it becomes a closed kinetic chain (CKC) movement. As a result, your joints are in a more stable position compared to an open kinetic chain (OKC) movement.

In this forward bend, the erector spinae and multifidus muscles work against the natural pull of gravity, allowing for a smooth transition without any jerks.

As you move into Uttanasana, the vertebral discs tend to shift backwards. Therefore, avoid this asana if you experience lower back issues.

I recommend maintaining an anterior pelvic tilt and avoiding rounding the back when transitioning from Samasthiti to Ardha Uttanasana. However, while transitioning from Ardha Uttanasana to Uttanasana, allow your spine to curve and assume a posterior pelvic tilt around 40–45 degrees of forward flexion originates from the lumbar spine, while 20–25 degrees originates from the thoracic spine. However, many people are instructed to bend solely from the lower back, which places excessive strain on the L4-L5 and L5-S1 vertebral junctions. These junctions are already highly susceptible to injury, and this misalignment can also increase the risk of hamstring strains.

Your neck is an integral part of the spine, so forcing it towards your knees can lead to neck problems. In Uttanasana, the cervical spine undergoes deep flexion, and repetitive practice may result in cervical spondylosis. Additionally, looking at your toes places unnecessary strain on your neck.

A useful tip to improve forward bending is to stretch the external rotators, ideally before practising, by internally rotating the hips—performing asanas like Matsyendrasana (Half Lord of the Fishes Pose) and Dandayamana Bhramanasana (Balancing Cat Pose/Bird Dog Pose). This also engages the hip's internal rotators—tensor fasciae latae, gluteus medius and minimus, and adductor longus. These muscles contribute significantly to pelvic stability, helping to distribute weight and movement more evenly.

Lastly, make sure to bend your knees slightly to relieve tension on the sciatic nerve. This will allow you to stretch your hamstring muscles more effectively. Otherwise, you risk overstretching the sciatic nerve.

Modifications

- **Regression:** Ensure you bend your knees if you experience excessive curving or load on your lower back. If you are not able to reach your toes, then grab your legs (or lower legs) either from the sides or behind.
- **Progression:** If you wish to progress into the Uttanasana, you can use yoga blocks and place your toes on the blocks while your heels are pressed into the ground (dorsiflexion). This will provide more stretch to your calf and hamstring muscles.

- **Prop Work:** One hack that could ease your Uttanasana practice is to engage your hip internal rotators with the help of a yoga block. To do so, fix a yoga block between your inner thighs, squeezing it gently with your thighs. This will engage your internal rotators, promoting a neutral pelvis and free movement of the spine in both directions.

Paschimottanasana (Seated Forward Bend)

Etymology: *Paschim* translates to West or back; *Uttana* means intense stretch; asana means posture

An asana that stretches the hamstrings, calves, and back muscles must be Paschimottanasana. It is one of the ancient asanas that can be traced back to the 13th century CE. It is depicted in hatha yoga scriptures, including Hatha Yoga Pradipika and Gheranda Samhita with numerous benefits. Hatha Yoga Pradipika says Paschimottanasana can help flatten the stomach, improve pranic energies (life force), and make us disease-free. However, for the maximum benefits, I suggest combining it with yogic mobility exercises, as doing so can fix

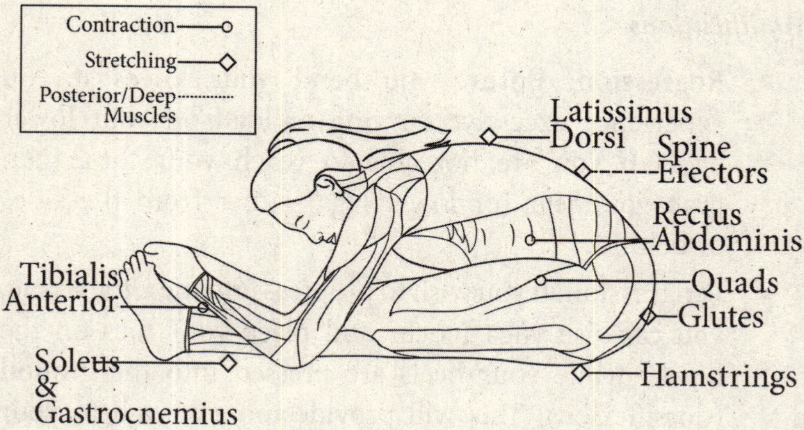

Paschimottanasana

your back, releasing tightness and allowing your hamstrings to release more efficiently.

Active Stretch: Trapezius and latissimus dorsi.

Asana Category	Targeted Area	Preparatory Yogic Practices
Beginner-friendly	Spine (flexion)	Dandasana (Staff Pose)
Forward-bending	Shoulder joints (flexion)	Matsyendrasana (Half Lord of Fishes Pose)
Hamstring stretch	Elbow joints (extension)	Uttanasana (Standing Forward Bend Pose)
Seated	Hip joints (flexion)	Marjaryasana and Bitilasana (Cat and Cow pose)
	Knee joints (extension)	
	Ankle joints (dorsiflexion)	

Technique:

a. Begin by assuming Dandasana.
b. On an inhale, lift your arms and stretch them completely over your head. Form a hook with your first two fingers. Meanwhile, lengthen your spine by tilting your hips forward as much as possible.
c. As you exhale, flex your torso forward without rounding your upper back. Keep your knees slightly bent.
d. Continuing the exhalation, once you have reached about a 60-degree angle, release the anterior tilt and allow your spine and hips to flex simultaneously. If possible, engage your core and quadriceps muscles for added support,

which will help release tension in the hamstrings, facilitating a deeper forward fold.

e. Inhale and, from the hook of your index and middle fingers, catch hold of your big toes—if your body allows. Otherwise, place your hands by the sides of your shins or hold your ankles.
f. Breathe normally and hold this position for 5 to 10 breaths, or as long as comfortable. Gently return to Dandasana. Repeat 3 to 5 times.

Benefits

- Stretches the entire back and rear leg muscles
- Releases tension from the back
- Helps those with a sedentary lifestyle
- Improves the flow of Prana energy—according to the hatha yoga scriptures
- Enhances reproductive health
- Tones the core
- Stimulates the internal smooth muscles, promoting healthy functioning of vital organs
- Calms the mind
- Relaxes the enteric nervous system

Common Mistakes to Avoid

- Hyperextending the knees
- Forcing the head to the knees
- A steep forward bend from your L4-L5 and L5-S1
- Gazing at the toes

Biomechanics

Have you ever wondered why Uttanasana feels easier than

Paschimottanasana? The key lies in the role of gravity. In Uttanasana, gravity assists the motion, allowing for a more natural contraction of the hip flexors, quadriceps, and abdominal muscles. In contrast, Paschimottanasana requires greater mechanical effort, as your body isn't aided by gravity in the same way. Additionally, in Paschimottanasana, your muscles are in contact with the ground, restricting the free movement of the hamstrings.

If your hamstrings are tight, your pelvis may not move as freely, leading to improper stretching of the spinal erectors. To address this, try myofascial release by rolling a tennis ball along the length of your hamstrings. This can help release tension and improve flexibility.

Engaging your hip internal rotators can significantly enhance your forward bends. You can achieve this in two ways—by stretching the external rotators of the hips before practice, or by placing a block between your thighs to activate the internal rotators. Many practitioners have tight external hip rotators due to everyday habits such as walking or sleeping positions. While walking, our legs naturally move into external rotation; otherwise, we'd walk like penguins! This tightness in the external rotators can place the pelvis in an awkward position. By working on the hip internal rotators, we can balance this external rotation and create smoother movement.

It is also common to hear yoga teachers say, 'Feel the stretch at the back of your knees—that's your hamstrings.' However, the hamstring muscles aren't actually located at the back of the knee. The tightness felt in that area is often due to the sciatic nerve, which runs through this region. Unlike muscles, nerves cannot be stretched. When the path of the sciatic nerve is restricted by surrounding muscles or tissues, it creates a sensation of tightness.

During forward bends, the abdominal and iliopsoas muscles (agonists) contract to initiate trunk flexion, which releases the spinal muscles and glutes (antagonists). Similarly, the quadriceps and tibialis anterior muscles (agonists) contract, causing the hamstrings, soleus, and gastrocnemius muscles (antagonists) to stretch.

When bending forward, the intervertebral discs protrude posteriorly towards the posterior longitudinal ligament (PLL). If the spinal discs are deformed, they can press against the spinal nerves, which pass through the spinal canal. For this reason, it's advisable to avoid this asana if you have any spinal condition.

Modifications

- **Prop Work:** Those who experience tightness in the pelvis or limited pelvic mobility should use a yoga blanket or block under their hips. This will increase the anterior pelvic tilt, allowing for easier movement.
- **Regression:** You can regress the pose by placing a soft yoga prop, like a blanket, underneath your knees.
- **Progression:** You can try PNF (proprioceptive neuromuscular facilitation) stretching. Contract your muscles for about 6 to 7 seconds, then allow them to relax for 3–4 seconds. This may help enhance the stretch.
- **Prop Work:** You can add a block between your thighs to engage your hip internal rotators. A rolled yoga blanket under your knees can also provide additional comfort while maintaining functionality.

Upavistha Konasana (Wide-Angle Seated Forward Bend)

Etymology: *Upavistha* translated to open or wide; *Kona* means angle; *Asana* means pose

The wide-angle seated forward bend can potentially reduce symptoms of menstrual distress (Oates 2017, 407–417). It also releases the muscles around the inner thighs and the groin area. Additionally, it involves bowing the head down, contributing to a sense of gratitude to Mother Earth. As it's said, a little gratitude goes a long way.

Active Stretch: Trapezius, erector spinae, quadratus lumborum, and transversospinalis.

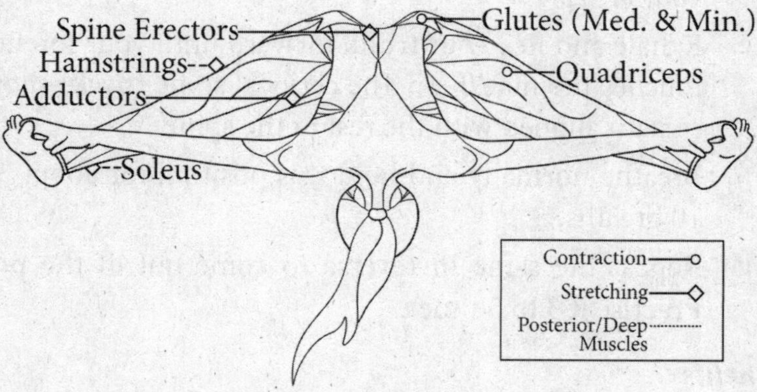

Upavistha Konasana

Asana Category	Targeted Area	Preparatory Yogic Practices
Sitting	Spine (flexion)	Balasana (Child's Pose)
Intermediate	Shoulder joints (flexion)	Paschimottanasana (Seated Forward Bend Pose)
Hip-opening	Elbow joints (extension)	Utkata Konasana (Goddess Pose)
Forward bend	Hip joints (abduction, external rotation)	
	Ankle joints (dorsiflexion)	

Technique:

a. Start by assuming Dandasana or sit with your legs extended in front of you.
b. From Dandasana, abduct your legs to the sides.
c. Assume a gentle anterior pelvic tilt by moving your hips slightly back.
d. Inhale and flex your shoulders overhead and fully extend your arms.
e. Exhale and flex your trunk forward until your forehead touches the mat/floor. The cervical spine (neck) should remain aligned with the rest of the spine.
f. Breathe normally and hold this position for about 3 to 10 breaths.
g. Repeat the same in reverse to come out of the pose. Practise it 3 to 5 times.

Benefits

- Stretches the adductor muscles (inner thighs)
- Activates the hip and hamstrings
- Expands the chest muscles
- Improves the respiratory system
- Helps with digestion
- Furthers kidney health
- Assists in the second trimester of pregnancy

Common Mistakes to Avoid

- Protruding your chin forward
- Hyperextending your knees
- Posterior pelvic tilt
- Rounding or arching your back

Biomechanics

The flexion of the trunk is facilitated by the iliopsoas and abdominal muscles (transverse abdominis and rectus abdominis). Meanwhile, the erector spinae, quadratus lumborum, and transversospinalis muscles engage while lengthening to gradually transition until we can rest. Here, an anterior pelvic tilt is recommended.

The trapezius muscle contracts to stabilise the scapulae and the neck, while the deltoid muscles lift the arms overhead and stabilise the shoulder joints.

The abduction of the hips is primarily supported by the gluteus medius, gluteus minimus, and tensor fasciae latae (TFL) muscles. Additionally, the quadriceps muscles extend the knee, while the semitendinosus and semimembranosus of the hamstring group stretch, along with the adductors.

The adductor muscles—located in the inner thighs—work as antagonists to the hip abductor muscles (agonists). Therefore, following the principle of reciprocal innervation, the adductor muscles are stretched when we assume the wide-angle pose.

Here, the peroneal muscles (longus and brevis) along with the tibialis anterior muscles contract, while the soleus and gastrocnemius muscles stretch.

In Upavistha Konasana, we can practise it as an open kinetic chain (OKC) movement or a closed kinetic chain (CKC) movement. To practise it as an OKC movement, you can keep your arms above the ground, engaging the erector spinae, quadratus lumborum, and transversospinalis muscles. In an OKC movement, the intensity of the asana will increase as the level of activation of various muscles increases. However, it is not recommended for individuals with spinal conditions. To practise it as a CKC movement, you should rest your arms on the mat/floor. Unlike an OKC movement, the erector spinae, quadratus lumborum, and transversospinalis muscles are stretched in a CKC movement, and these stretches are comparatively mild.

Modifications

- **Regression:** If you cannot completely flex your trunk forward, place your arms in front of you and adjust according to your convenience.
- **Progression:** If you wish to progress into this asana, aim for a complete middle split. However, keep it within your comfort range and progress gradually.
- **Prop Work:** You can also use props like yoga blocks and bolsters in front to limit the flexion of the trunk.
- **Yin Yoga:** For yin yoga, you can add a blanket under your sit bones (ischial tuberosity) to increase your anterior pelvic tilt. Additionally, you can add rolled blankets under your knees to restrict discomfort.

11

Open Heart, Open Mind: Exploring Backward Bending Asanas

Back-bending asanas help to extend our spine. In today's digital age, our spines tend to slouch more than ever. To address this issue, yoga therapists often recommend back-bending asanas. However, it's important to be aware that backbends can put pressure on the facet joints (intervertebral joints). In this chapter, we will explore back-bending asanas and how to overcome some of the challenges associated with them.

Hasta Uttanasana (Standing Backward Bend Pose)

Etymology: *Hasta* means hand; *Uttana* translates to intense stretch; and *Asana* means pose.

Since our initial development, we had a slouching stance; therefore, our bodies have an affinity for slouching. This permits various forces to act on our spine. Hasta Uttanasana, a beginner-friendly back-bending pose, can counteract these forces. It offers a nice extension to the spine and focuses on the co-contraction of the spinal and abdominal muscles.

Active Stretch: Rectus abdominis, transverse abdominis, quadriceps (rectus femoris), and iliopsoas.

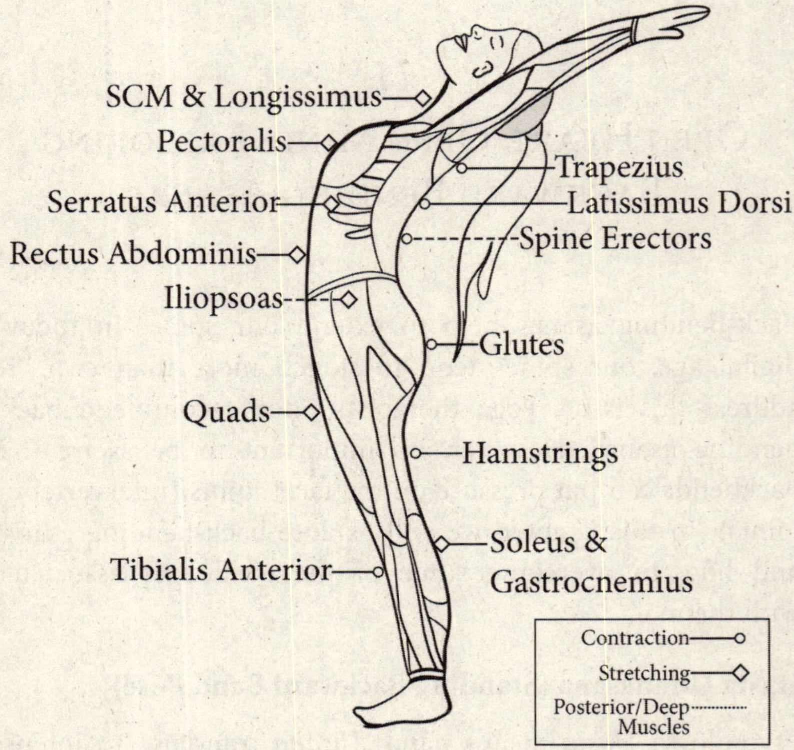

Hasta Uttanasana

Asana Category	Targeted Area	Preparatory Yogic Practices
Backbend Standing -	Spine (extension), chest/heart opening Shoulder joints (flexion) Elbow joints (extension) Hip joints (extension) Knee joints (extension) Ankle joints (neutral)	Samasthiti (Equal Pose) Tadasana (Palm Tree Pose) Urdhva Hastasana (Upward Salute Pose) -

Technique:

a. Begin with Tadasana or Samisthiti. Draw your legs shoulder-width apart.
b. Inhale and lift your arms over your head.
c. As you continue to inhale, squeeze your hip muscles and bend backwards to a comfortable point. You can focus on opening the chest.
d. Breathe normally and engage your core without interrupting the flow of your breath.
e. Continue to breathe normally and hold this position for 3 to 10 breaths for 2 to 5 rounds.
f. Repeat the instructions in reverse to come out of the pose.

Benefits

- Activates several muscles, including spine erectors and other back muscles
- Counters the effects of a rounded upper back and shoulders
- Gives room to the diaphragm
- Improves the respiration capacity
- Opens the chest and heart
- Alleviates tightness of the upper back

Common Mistakes to Avoid

- Difficulty breathing or holding your breath
- Steep backbends—in extreme cases, it can also lead to dizziness
- Improper/poor muscle engagement

- Handing your neck freely
- Flexing your knees

Biomechanics

It is a good idea to either work on your hip internal rotators before practising Hasta Uttanasana or exhaust your hip external rotators. Both methods should make the backward extension of the spine easier.

In Hasta Uttanasana, the abdominal muscles contract while lengthening to sustain the motion against gravity, whereas the erector spinae and transversospinalis muscles (multifidus) contract concentrically.

In the upper back (thoracic spine), the trapezius muscles contract with the spine erectors, releasing the pectoralis muscles. Additionally, the co-activation of abdominal and back muscles counters the compression over the facet joints (spinal joints). Thus, ensure you activate your abdominal muscles sufficiently without compromising your breath.

The co-contraction of the gluteal muscles (hip extensors) and iliopsoas (hip flexors) is also crucial, as it stabilises the pelvis—especially the lumbosacral (L5-S1) joint—and prevents excessive force from being transferred to the sacroiliac (SI) joint.

As we move into deeper bends, more force is directed towards the lower segment of the spine (T12-S1 vertebrae), causing deep compression. Therefore, maintain a gradual and even spine extension.

Similarly, if you bend your neck or back or try to look upwards, the vertebral joints of the neck will also compress, which can result in neck pain.

It is worth noting that the cervical spine has a unique structure where the transverse foramen carries the carotid arteries to the head. If these arteries are obstructed, you might feel dizzy. Giddiness can also arise from rapid changes in blood pressure. Thus, I recommend keeping the neck aligned with the rest of the spine, staying hydrated, and breathing well.

Modifications

- **Regression:** You can always regress into the asana by opting for a mild back bend.
- **Progression:** If you wish to experience more stretch, you can practise Ardha Chakrasana (Half Wheel Pose). Place your hands on your waist and bend further back while engaging your core and hip muscles as best as you can.
- **Prop Work:** You can add a block between your thighs to prevent the external rotation of your legs. Doing so will decompress your lower back.

Bhujangasana (Cobra Pose)

Etymology: Bhujanga translates to cobra; asana means posture.

If you ask me about one of the best asanas for spinal ailments, I recommend Bhujangasana. It is named after the cobra, as it resembles its hood. The special thing about it is its ability to prevent spinal ailments, making it widely recommended by doctors, physiotherapists, and yoga teachers. It is also a part of the traditional Surya Namaskar and comes in the sequence at the 7th spot.

Active Stretch: Pectoralis, biceps brachii, iliopsoas, and transverse abdominis.

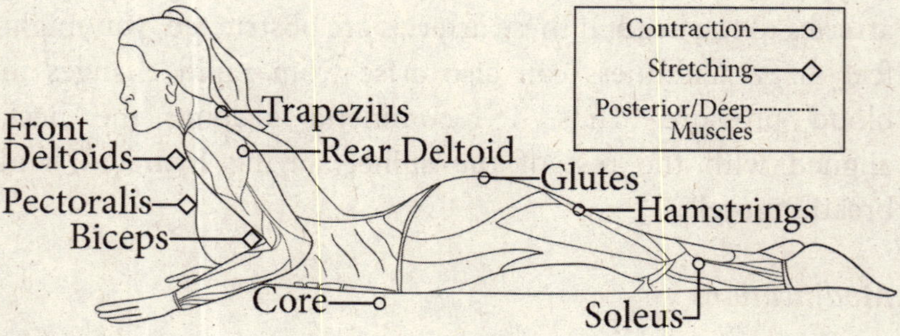

Bhujangasana

Asana Category	Targeted Area	Preparatory Yogic Practices
Backbend	Spine (extension)	Ardh Bhujangasana (Baby Cobra Pose)
Beginner-friendly	Upper cervical spine (flexion)	Salamba Bhujangasana (Sphinx Pose)
Prone-lying	Shoulder joints (extension)	
	Elbow joints (flexion)	
	Hip joints (extension)	
	Knee joints (extension)	

Technique:

a. Assume a lying position on your stomach.
b. Your legs must be shoulder-width apart, with your toes pointing outwards.
c. Place your palms underneath your shoulders, ensuring a strong grip of your fingers on the yoga mat.
d. Inhale and gradually extend your elbows while keeping them close to the sides. Lift your upper body only until the navel (Manipura or solar plexus chakra).
e. Breathe normally and tuck your chin in, gaze forward. Roll your shoulders up, back, down, and retract your

shoulder plates. Focus on opening the chest as much as possible.

f. As you continue to breathe normally, hold this posture for 3 to 10 breaths with proper muscle engagement.
g. Remain calm and mindful throughout.
h. Exhale and bend your elbows, relaxing your entire body in the prone position.
i. Practise 3 to 5 times a day.

Benefits

- Helps prevent backache—in several cases, it also relieves existing back pain
- Helps strengthen arm muscles
- Aligns the spinal column
- Improves the flexibility of your spine
- Helps with type 2 diabetes, digestion, etc.
- Aids in respiratory health
- Opens the chest and anterior shoulders

Common Mistakes to Avoid

- Gazing upwards
- Complete extension of your elbows
- Elevating your shoulders
- Joining your legs, especially if you suffer from spinal ailments

Biomechanics

In Bhujangasana, it is critical to maintain a gradual backbend and allow the thoracic spine to participate. This approach improves the mobility and rhythm of the entire spine, as opposed to focusing on the already overused L1-S1 segment of the lower spine. If the backbend is initiated from the L1-S1 segment, an injury could occur due to compressive forces.

The core muscles act as natural stabilisers to safeguard your lower spine, helping to minimise compression and loading.

Avoid fully extending the elbows, as this places strain on the L4-L5 and L5-S1 sections of the spine, as well as the elbow joints. This also leads to poor engagement of the triceps and biceps brachii muscles.

Looking upwards puts the lower cervical spine in flexion and the upper cervical in extension. However, to keep the cervical spine healthy, one should do the reverse—the lower cervical spine should be extended, and the upper cervical flexed.

The cobra pose activates the entire posterior chain of muscles, while the anterior chain stretches. Additionally, focus on engaging the gluteal muscles while medially rotating the legs, as this creates more space for the spine.

From the early stages of embryonic development, we are accustomed to a rounded spine, and this tendency remains evident in our everyday posture. To counterbalance this, backbends should be practised regularly.

Since the posterior longitudinal ligaments (PLLs) of the spine are weaker than the anterior longitudinal ligaments (ALLs), practising backbends more often can help prevent injury.

The imbibition phenomenon supplies resources to the spine and surrounding tissue, but it relies on spinal movements. Thus, spinal mobility is essential for maintaining a healthy body.

Moreover, spinal extension is facilitated by the erector spinae, transversospinalis, and trapezius muscles. The serratus anterior and trapezius muscles also stabilise the scapulae.

Practitioners often move their elbows outward, which typically indicates short supinators or weak pronators. In such cases, working on wrist mobility exercises can be highly beneficial.

Modifications

- **Variation-I/Regression:** If you experience any back-related ailment, you can regress into the Ardha Bhujangasana (Half Cobra) practice. In this pose, lift the chest only about 6 to 10 inches off the ground. Doing this will gently stretch the chest and shoulder muscles while engaging the back muscles.
- **Variation-II/Modification:** Individuals who experience backaches must practise Bhujangasana with legs shoulder-width apart, as it provides more room to the pelvis and creates a more stable base. This also helps overcome hyperextension or compression of the back.
- **Progression:** I would not suggest going into a steep backbend. However, if you have good spinal mobility in the thoracic spine segment, you can experiment by extending your elbows slightly, without complete extension.
- **Prop Work:** You can fold and place a yoga blanket or towel underneath your waist to curb discomfort.
    - Additionally, I recommend choosing Bhujangasana over Urdhva Mukha Svanasana (Upward Facing Dog Pose), as Bhujangasana is more stable. While both are similar, they offer valuable differences.

Setu Bandhasana (Bridge Pose)

Etymology: *Setu* means bridge; *Bandha* means noose or formation; *Asana* means posture.

If you wish to improve sexual, urinary, and pelvic floor muscle health, Setu Bandhasana can be an apt choice. It strengthens your lower body, including the glutes, thighs, and calf muscles, while also improving their aesthetics.

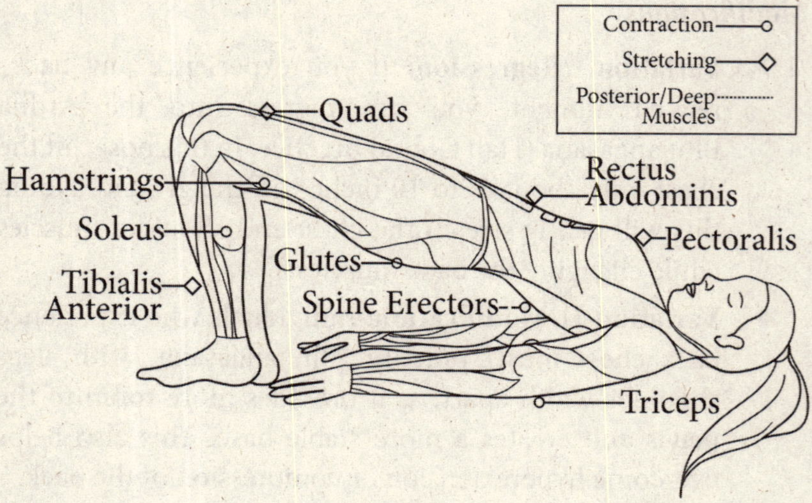

Setu Bandhasana

Asana Category	Targeted Area	Preparatory Yogic Practices
Backbend	Cervical (flexion), thoracic and lumbar spine (extension)	Ustrasana (Camel Pose)
Chest Opening	Shoulder joints (extension)	Dwi Pada Viparita Dandasana (Upward Facing Two-Foot Staff Pose)
Beginner-friendly	Elbow joints (extension)	Marjaryasana and Bitilasana (Cat and Cow mobility)
Upside-Down/ Inversion	Hip joints (extension)	
Leg Intensive	Knee joints (flexion)	
Supine Lying	Ankle joints (neutral)	

Additionally, it stretches the neck, chest, and abdominal muscles. It is primarily categorised as a chest opening, glute-strengthening, and inverted asana.

Active Stretch: Pectoralis, rectus abdominis, transverse abdominis, quadriceps, and TFL.

Technique:

a. Start from a reclining position or Shavasana (Corpse Pose). Keep your arms by the side of your body with palms facing downwards.
b. Bend your knees and place the heels directly under your knees while maintaining a hip-width gap between your legs.
c. Inhale and lift your chest, waist, and hips simultaneously off the floor. Generate a push from your heels and arms.
d. Breathe normally and keep your chest to a preferable height. Keep your thighs almost parallel to the floor and clasp your fingers.
e. Continue to breathe normally, tuck your tailbone in and engage your hip muscles as best as you can. Tuck your chin in.
f. Breathe normally and hold this pose for about 10 to 30 seconds.
g. Exhale and relax comfortably by bringing your body back to the mat.

Benefits

- Helps co-contract the front and back torso muscles
- Fortifies the upper and lower spine, preventing damage.
- Opens the tight chest muscles

- Activates the glutes
- Prevents the dead butt syndrome
- Facilitates better hip mobility
- Releases tight hip flexor muscles
- Improves the ability to bend backwards
- Enhances our respiratory performance
- Strengthens the spinal muscles
- Can alleviate varicose veins

Common Mistakes to Avoid

- Burdening the neck
- Lifting your heels off the ground
- Externally rotating the legs
- Excessively extending the knees outwards or inwards

Biomechanics

To engage the muscles adequately, press your heels down. This will enhance the activation of the hamstring and soleus muscles. Clasping your fingers stretches the serratus anterior muscles.

To generate lift, the spinal erectors, gluteus maximus, hamstrings, soleus, and gastrocnemius muscles contract in synergy. Meanwhile, the abdominal, iliopsoas, and quadriceps muscles stretch while stabilising the movement.

The trapezius and rhomboid muscles stabilise the scapulae, helping to open the chest area. Activation of the gluteus maximus can compress the pelvis, as it performs both hip extension and external rotation. To mitigate this, activating the hip internal rotators, TFL, gracilis, gluteus medius, and minimus muscles before practising this asana can be beneficial.

Lastly, the posterior deltoid muscles help extend the shoulders, while the triceps muscles extend the elbows.

Modifications

- **Regression:** If you experience discomfort or wish to regress in the pose, I recommend keeping the body gradually aligned from head to knees, without lifting the waist (or hips) too high.
- **Progression:** To advance in the Bridge Pose, I suggest squeezing the gluteal and core muscles to the maximum extent for 7 seconds, then relaxing for 3 seconds (using contract-relax stretching). This will further release your muscles.
- **Prop Work:** If you'd like to make Setu Bandhasana more relaxing, place a yoga block under your lower back. This will provide support and make the posture more comfortable.
- **Prop Work:** Wrapping your legs with a yoga belt may also prevent external rotation of the hips.

Chakrasana/Urdhva Dhanurasana (Wheel Pose)

Etymology: *Urdhva* translates to upward; *Dhanura* means bow; *Chakra* means wheel; asana translates to posture or pose.

If you wish to improve the mobility of your spine, shoulders, and hips, Chakrasana can be a great option. The name 'Wheel Pose' is derived from the Sanskrit name 'Chakrasana', whereas Urdhva Dhanurasana (Upside Down Bow Pose) is derived from the Ashtanga Vinyasa sequence. The Wheel Pose is an intermediate to advanced pose. Therefore, I suggest practising Chakrasana only when you have been performing asanas like Bhujangasana (Cobra Pose), Salamba Bhujangasana (Sphinx

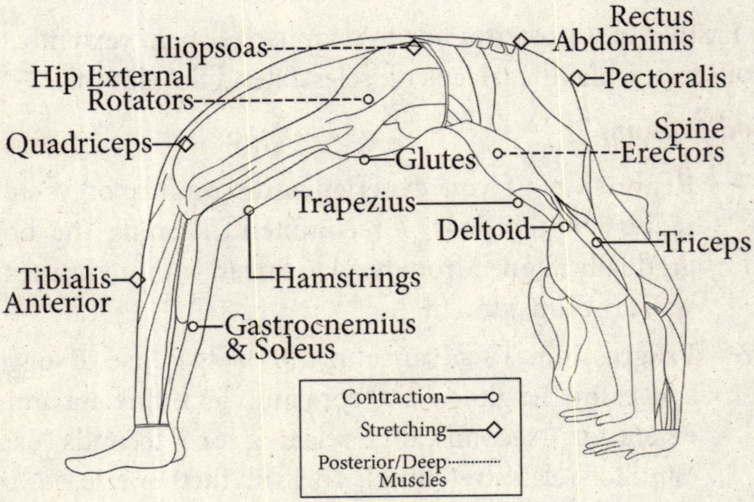

Chakrasana

Asana Category	Targeted Area	Preparatory Yogic Practices
Intermediate	Spine (extension)	Dhanurasana (Bow Pose)
Backbend	Shoulder joints (flexion)	Bhujangasana (Cobra Pose)
Chest/heart-opening	Elbow joints (extension)	Ustrasana (Camel Pose)
Upside-down/ inversion	Wrist joints (extension)	Setu Bandhasana (Bridge Pose)
Strengthening	Hip joints (extension	-
-	Knee joints (extension)	-

Pose), Dhanurasana (Bow Pose), etc, for a while. Lastly, remember that it also relies greatly on the mobility of your shoulder joints.

Active Stretch: Rectus abdominis, transverse abdominis, pectoralis, iliopsoas, serratus anterior, biceps brachii, quadriceps, and latissimus dorsi.

Technique:

a. Assume a reclining position or Shavasana (Corpse Pose). Keep your legs hip-width apart and arms shoulder-width apart.
b. Bend your knees and bring them close to your buttocks. Similarly, flex your shoulders and elbows so that you can place your palms on the floor by the side of your crown.
c. Inhale and gently tuck your chin in and lift your head off the mat, ensuring your shoulders remain almost parallel to your palms. Your arms should generate and initiate the lift, not the legs.
d. Continue inhaling and press your heels down on the mat to generate additional lift from your calf and hamstring muscles.
e. Breathe normally and engage your core and gluteus muscles as best as possible.
f. Continue to breathe normally and hold this position for about 3 to 10 breaths.
g. Exhale and gently lower your body with complete control and come back on the mat. Repeat this 2 to 5 times.

Benefits

- Prevents spinal injuries
- Can improve spinal health
- Tones and stretches the abdominal, shoulder, and chest muscles
- Can improve lung capacity by expanding the lungs
- Believed to activate the Anahata chakra (Heart chakra)

- Strengthens the hamstring muscles, spine erectors, and pelvic stabiliser muscles

Common Mistakes to Avoid

- A steep backbend
- Bending your elbows
- Moving your toes outwards
- Initiating the lift from your legs

Biomechanics

In Chakrasana, initiate the lift from your arms rather than your legs. Otherwise, the strong activation of the leg muscles causes the head to move away from the arms, reducing the likelihood of reaching the peak pose. However, immobile shoulders could also result in a similar outcome.

Due to tightness in the external hip rotators, most yoga practitioners are likely to externally rotate their hip joints. This creates discomfort in the pelvis, forcing the spine to bear more compressive forces. I recommend engaging the internal hip rotators, such as the gluteus medius and minimus muscles, as doing so alleviates compressive forces on the spine and allows for a proper range of motion.

Similarly, to stabilise your shoulders and scapulae, you can externally rotate your arms. The infraspinatus, teres minor, deltoid, and triceps brachii muscles also contribute to shoulder stability.

In Chakrasana, the iliopsoas stretches while the glutes extend the hips, resisting gravity.

It is always advisable to prioritise the underused thoracic spine over the overused lumbar and cervical spine.

Here, the abdominal and chest muscles act against gravity while lengthening. Meanwhile, the muscles of the back, such as the erector spinae, transversospinalis, quadratus lumborum, and trapezius, help stabilise the torso and pelvis, working closely with the abdominal and chest muscles to maintain the movement. Overall, this asana activates the entire posterior chain of muscles. Moreover, the hamstrings and quadriceps contract in tandem to extend the legs.

When we properly distribute weight between the toes and heels, they activate two powerful posterior leg muscles—the soleus and gastrocnemius.

Lastly, here, the abdominal and back muscles co-contract to counteract gravity.

Modifications

- **Regression:** To regress, you can try Ardha Chakrasana (Half Wheel Pose).
- **Progression:** Progression in Wheel Pose is not recommended for many individuals. However, if you still wish to attempt it, try practising Purna Chakrasana (Advanced Wheel Pose). In this variation, you bring the palms and heels closer together, completing the wheel formation.
- **Prop Work:** You can place a yoga block between your thighs to activate your hip internal rotators, which will counteract the hip external rotators. The external rotator muscles compress the pelvis, which is undesirable.

Raja Kapotasana (King Pigeon Pose) and Eka Pada Kapotasana (Pigeon Pose)

If you are looking for an asana that eases stress from the hip muscles and offers a mild backbend, look no further than Kapotasana. It primarily emphasises hip-opening and can be easily practised by beginners. It also comes with an advanced variation, Raja Kapotasana (King Pigeon Pose or Royal Pigeon Pose), which is a much more intense backbend.

I strongly recommend adding Kapotasana to your hip-opening yoga sequences and pre-practice stretches.

Active Stretch: Pectoralis, tibialis anterior, intercostals, serratus anterior, gluteus medius and minimus (ipsilateral).

Asana Category	Targeted Area	Preparatory Yogic Practices
Beginner-friendly/ advanced	Spine (extension)	Agni Stambhasana (Fire Log Pose)
Hip-opening	Shoulder joints (flexion)	Sucirandhrasana (Eye the Needle Pose)
Chest/heart-opening	Elbow joints (flexion)	Bhujangasana (Cobra Pose)
-	Pelvis (anterior pelvic tilt)	Gomukhasana (Cow Facing Pose)
-	Hip joint (flexion) (external rotation) (ipsilateral)	-
-	Hip joint (extension) (contralateral)	-
-	Knee joints (flexion) (contralateral extension in kapotasana)	-
-	Ankle joints (plantar flexion)	-

Kapotasana (Pigeon Pose)

Etymology: *Kapot* translates to pigeon; *Asana* means pose.

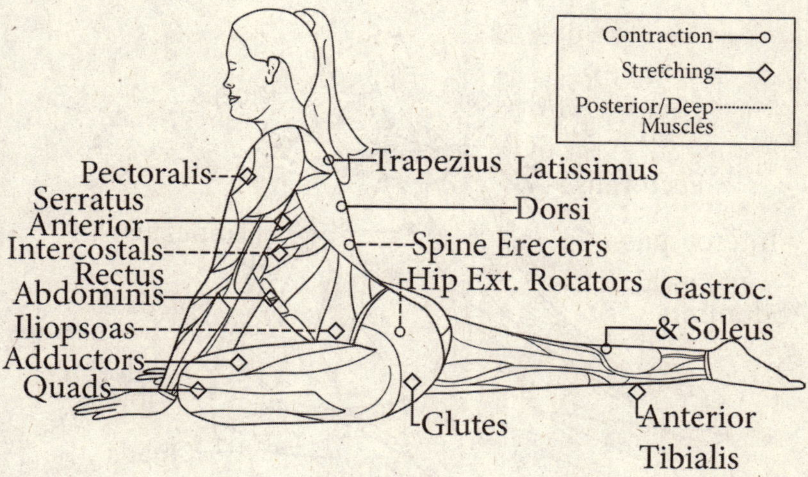

Kapotasana

Technique

a. Assume Bhramanasana (Table Top Pose).
b. From Bhramanasana, externally rotate and flex your right knee (ipsilateral) and place it in the front. The right heel should be next to the left side of your pelvis.
c. Extend your left leg (contralateral) back. Additionally, ensure you can place your pelvis on the mat. Try to square your hips to your best.
d. Inhale and bring your arms close to your body in front to gently stretch backwards.

Raja Kapotasana (King Pigeon Pose)

Etymology: *Raja* means king; *Kapot* translates to pigeon; *Asana* means posture.

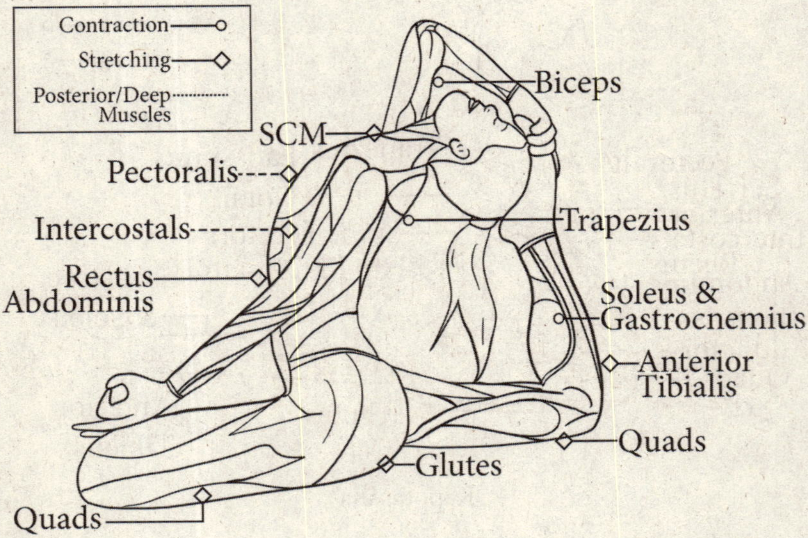

Raja Kapotasana

Technique:

a. Inhale and, from the Pigeon Pose, allow your entire torso to bend backwards. If you manage to keep your left knee in the centre, then flexing the left knee will bring the heel close to your head.breathe normally and, with both hands (right followed by left), catch hold of the left big toe.

b. Continue to breathe normally and keep your spine comfortable. Hold this position for 3 to 10 breaths or what your body allows.

c. Repeat this 3 to 5 times on each side.

Benefits

- Can relieve deep gluteal syndrome
- Releases deep pelvic muscles
- Helps mobilise the hip joints
- Stretches the chest and abdominal muscles
- Helps improve the respiratory system
- Releases tension from the upper back
- Provides a gentle extension for the back
- Can prevent backache
- Strengthens the shoulders, entire back, and hip muscles

Common Mistakes to Avoid

- Malalignment of your neck from the rest of the spine
- Lifting your pelvis off the floor
- Tilting to any side
- Jerky movements
- Moving your bent knee beneath or away from the pelvis
- Straining your arms
- Overstretching
- Any rotation of your extended leg
- Practising without adequate supervision

Biomechanics

Moving your cervical spine (neck) into deep extension while the rest of your spine is in mild extension should be avoided. Ideally, the front hip flexes and externally rotates, while the rear hip extends with a slight internal rotation.

Often, yoga practitioners tend to lift the pelvis while aiming for the backbend. It is worth noting that the pigeon postures are more focused on hip opening than the backbend. Therefore, aim for better hip opening, and chest opening will follow.

In Pigeon Pose, we activate the entire posterior chain of muscles, including the erector spinae, transversospinalis, quadratus lumborum, hamstrings, trapezius, latissimus dorsi, gastrocnemius, and soleus muscles. Meanwhile, most of the muscles from the anterior chain are stretched, including the abdominal muscles (rectus abdominis and transverse abdominis), quadriceps, pectoralis, tibialis anterior, external and internal intercostal muscles, and serratus anterior muscles.

Core muscles act as natural stabilisers to safeguard your lower spine, particularly the transverse abdominis and transversospinalis, which work together to support the lumbar spine and minimise compression and loading. The trapezius muscles contract with the spine erectors, while the quadratus lumborum facilitates the backbend and stabilises the spine and pelvis, stretching the chest and abdominal muscles.

The ipsilateral leg can be externally rotated by the iliopsoas and hip external rotator muscles (piriformis, gemellus, and obturator internus). To slightly abduct the ipsilateral leg, the sartorius, gluteus medius, and minimus muscles act in synergy, while the ipsilateral adductor muscles are stretched.

The rear leg requires the contraction of several muscles to sustain the motion, including the gluteal muscles, hamstrings, gastrocnemius, and soleus. Meanwhile, the iliopsoas, quadriceps, and tibialis anterior muscles are stretched.

Lastly, in Pigeon Pose, the triceps contract to extend the elbows. In King Pigeon Pose, the biceps contract to bend the elbows.

Modifications

- **Regression:** If you find the backbend too intense, you can opt for a standard Kapotasana or Kapotasana with flexed elbows.
- **Progression:** If you wish to progress into Raja Kapotasana, engage your core muscles without disrupting your breath.
- **Progression—Prop Work:** To transition from Kapotasana to Raja Kapotasana, start by placing yoga blocks or a bolster under your arms. This will increase the backward extension of your spine.
- **Prop Work:** You can also use a yoga strap or belt around your shin or ankle and slowly pull the strap to transition from Pigeon Pose to King Pigeon Pose.
- **Counterpose:** After practising this asana, you can recline forward by flexing your trunk and resting here.
- **Yin Yoga:** In yin yoga, you can fill the gap between your pelvis and the mat with a yoga blanket or bolster. Place another bolster in front. To practise yin yoga Kapotasana, support your forearms or arms on the bolster. For the forward-bending variation of Kapotasana, you can hug the bolster.

12

Vulnerability and Strength: Heart-Opening Asanas for Growth

Heart-opening asanas focus on expanding the chest and are closely linked with the Anahata chakra, or the heart chakra, which governs our emotions. While heart-openers and backbends share many similarities, the key distinction is that most backbends primarily target the lumbar spine (lower back), whereas the heart-opening asanas target the thoracic spine (mid-back). In this chapter, we will explore how opening the heart can release negative emotions, inviting positive energy to flow in.

Gomukhasana (Cow Face Pose)

Etymology: *Go* (or *Gau*) means cow: *Mukh* means face; *Asana* means posture.

Gomukhasana is a versatile asana that stretches hard-to-reach muscles in our body. It stretches our shoulder, upper back, glutes, and deep hip muscles. Some of these muscles are seldom stretched but overused. Due to its effectiveness, Gomukhasana is often suggested for various sports enthusiasts and athletes. It also helps ease emotional baggage, making us feel rejuvenated.

Active Stretch: Tibialis anterior, intercostals, glutes, hip external rotators, and pectoralis.

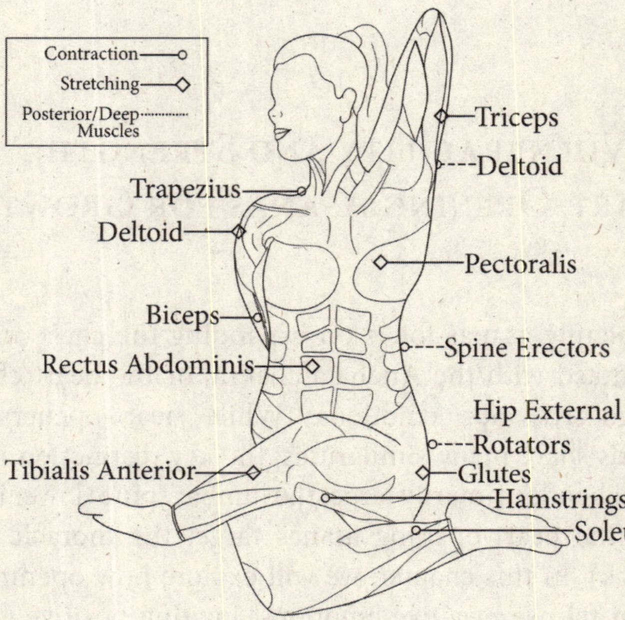

Gomukhasana

Asana Category	Targeted Area	Preparatory Yogic Practices
Beginner-friendly	Spine (axial extension)	Sukhasana (Easy Pose)
Shoulder stretch	Shoulder joints (flexion) (internal rotation) (ipsilateral)	Agni Stambhasana (Fire Log Pose)
Hip-opener	Shoulder joints (extension) (internal rotation) (contralateral)	Kapotasana (Pigeon Pose)
Seated	Wrist joints (flexion)	
	Hip joints (external rotation) (flexion) (adduction)	
	Knee joints (flexion)	
	Ankle joints (plantar flexion)	

Technique:

a. Assume Dandasana or sit with your legs extended in front of you.
b. Bend your right knee and place it in the middle of your body.
c. Now, bend your left knee and stack it on the top of your right knee. Let your toes face opposite sides.
d. Inhale, lift your left arm and rotate it internally, and then flex your right elbow and place it on your left scapula blade.
e. Exhale and rotate your right arm internally, flexing it from the underside, and try to catch hold of the fingers of the right arm.
f. Breathe normally and keep your spine long. Hold this position for about 5 to 10 breaths.
g. Repeat this 3 to 5 times on each side.

Benefits

- Stretches the shoulders, chest, and abdominal muscles
- Extends the hip external rotators
- Helps overcome deep gluteal syndrome
- Therapeutic for our spinal health
- Strengthens the adductor muscles
- Activates the hip internal rotators
- Mobilises the shoulders
- Improves rotator cuff muscle health
- Can improve respiration
- Enhances digestion

- Promotes spinal health
- Improves the forward and backward bending asanas

Common Mistakes to Avoid

- Hunching or rounding the back
- Straining the knees
- Jutting the chin forward
- Placing your arms in an uncomfortable position
- Arching your back
- Forcing yourself into the pose

Biomechanics

The gluteus medius and minimus, tensor fascia lata, sartorius, and adductor longus muscles primarily contribute the internal hip rotation. Meanwhile, the opposing muscles—hip external rotator muscles stretch, such as gluteus maximus, piriformis, gemellus, and obturator internus muscles.

While practising Gomukhasana, both of your arms should internally rotate. However, many people struggle to clasp their hands due to the immediate internal rotation of the bottom arm. To understand this better, when we internally rotate, the scapula blade moves away from the midline (abduction) and hinders the motion. Whereas, if you externally rotate the shoulder, your scapula will rest against the rib, giving you more room to move your arm. To put it into perspective, first, externally rotate your lower arm, bring it to the back, internally rotate it, and flex the elbow. In most situations, you should be able to reach your arms.

The flexion of the knees comes from the hamstring muscles and adduction from the adductor muscles. The gastrocnemius and soleus muscles plantarflex the ankle joints.

The erector spinae, transversospinalis, trapezius, and quadratus lumborum act in synergy to keep the spine erect. This leads to gentle stretch of the chest muscles.

To prevent any injury, keep the scapula stable and monitor the motion of the knees properly. If necessary, restrict the motion with the appropriate yoga props.

Modifications

- **Regression:** Grab a yoga belt or strap and progress until you can hold your hands.
- **Progression:** To progress, you can further stretch your arms.
- **Prop Work:** You can add a yoga blanket under your sit bones to prevent your back from rounding. You can also use yoga blocks under your ankles to limit your leg movements to regress.
- **Yin Yoga (Reclining Gomukhasana):** To practise reclining Gomukhasana, you can place a folded yoga blanket under your shin to limit your hip external rotation beyond your comfort. Additionally, place a yoga bolster in front to make it comfortable.

Uttana Shishosana (Extended Puppy Pose)

Etymology: *Uttana* translates to intense stretch; *Shisho* means puppy; *Asana* means posture.

If you need an asana to ease the built-up tension in your entire body, I highly recommend Uttana Shishosana. It helps improve the overall body posture and has combinational properties of Balaṣana (Child Pose), Adho Mukha Svanasana (Downward Facing Dog Pose), and Ardha Pincha Mayurasana (Dolphin Pose). Moreover, it is also believed to be linked with the Anahata chakra which is believed to be located at the heart centre. Yin yoga chest-opening sessions are incomplete without the Extended Puppy Pose.

Active Stretch: Glutes, latissimus dorsi, transverse abdominis, and quadriceps.

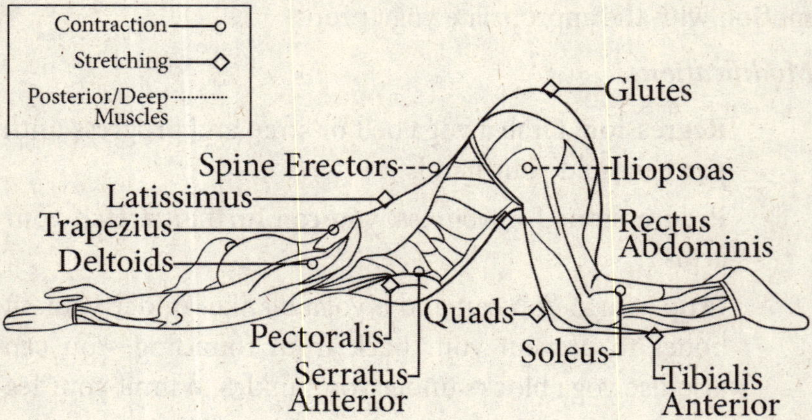

Uttana Shishosana

Asana Category	Targeted Area	Preparatory Yogic Practices
Chest/heart-opening	Spine (extension)	Balasana (Child's Pose)
Forward bend	Shoulder joints (flexion)	Adho Mukha Svanasana (Downward Facing Dog Pose)
Kneeling	Hip joints (flexion)	Ardha Pincha Mayurasana (Dolphin Pose)
Arm stretch	Knee joints (flexion)	-
Inversion upside-down	Ankle joints (plantar flexion)	-

Technique:

a. Begin in Bhramanasana (Table Top Pose), positioning your knees directly under your hips and your wrists under your shoulders. Ensure there is a hip-width distance between your knees and a shoulder-width distance between your hands. Point your toes outwards.
b. Inhale and stretch your hands forward until your forehead touches the mat.
c. Breathe normally and hold this position for about 10 breaths.
d. To return, slowly bring your palms under your shoulders and gently lift your body, coming out of the pose with control.

Benefits

- Extends the spine and releases tightness from the surrounding tissues
- Prevents rounding of the upper back
- Can ease built-up tension from the upper back
- Helps relax after a hectic day at work
- Can help activate the Anahata chakra (heart chakra).
- Improves the flexibility of the upper back
- Can improve respiration
- Can enhance the range of motion of the shoulders

Common Mistakes to Avoid

- Leaning too far backwards or forward
- Extensive anterior pelvic tilt
- Gazing forward

Biomechanics

Here, the spinal erectors, trapezius, and transverse abdominis muscles work together to keep the spine extended against the pull of gravity, while the rectus abdominis muscle stretches.

Press into the ground with your palm flexor muscles to activate your back muscles and open your chest further.

The trapezius and serratus anterior muscles stabilise the scapulae. Keeping your chin slightly tucked in will help maintain a neutral cervical curve.

The iliopsoas muscles flex the hip joints while the gluteal muscles stretch. The hamstring muscles bend the knees, and the quadriceps muscles ensure the knees remain at a 90-degree angle. The gastrocnemius and soleus muscles plantarflex the toes, stretching the tibialis anterior muscles.

Modifications

- **Regression:** You can practise this pose with the help of wall support. You can also use a yoga bolster to support your upper body.
- **Progression:** If you want to deepen the pose, you can move into an anterior pelvic tilt and lower your chest towards the ground, which will also open up your chest.
- **Prop Work:** To support your head, place a yoga blanket or block in front.
- **Yin Yoga:** You can add a yoga bolster vertically between your chest. Doing so will allow you to hold this asana for some time while experiencing mild stretches.

Ustrasana (Camel Pose)

Etymology: *Ustra* translates to camel; *Asana* means pose or posture.

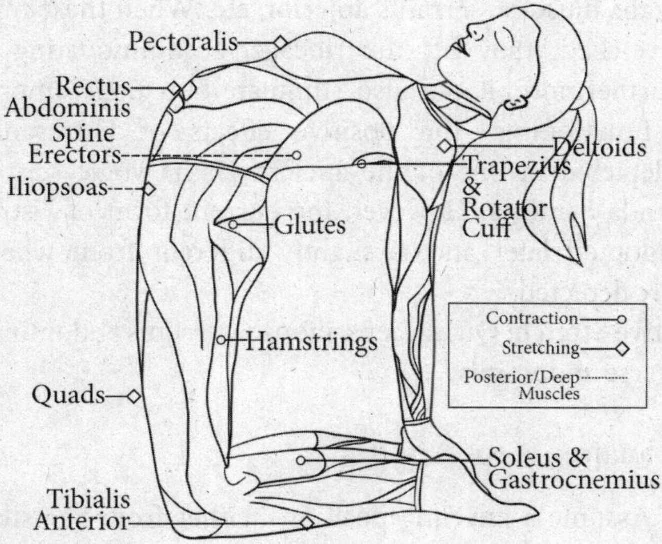

Ustrasana

Asana Category	Targeted Area	Preparatory Yogic Practices
Backbend	Spine (extension)	Matsyasana (Fish Pose)
Chest/heart-opening	Shoulder joints (extension)	Hastottanasana (Standing Back Bend Pose)
Kneeling	Neck (extension)	Vajrasana (Thunderbolt Pose)
-	Hip joints (extension)	-
-	Knee joints (flexion)	-
-	Ankle joints (plantar flexion)	-

Ustrasana can improve one's lung capacity (tidal volume) by opening the chest and easing the accessory muscles of respiration, such as the external and internal intercostals, pectoralis muscles, serratus anterior, etc. When these muscles are stretched, they lift the ribcage, accommodating more air. Furthermore, it can also stimulate our lungs, improving their functioning. The positive effects of Ustrasana are also depicted in one of the ancient Hatha yogic scriptures, Gheranda Samhita. However, the current form of Ustrasana was adopted later and is slightly different from what was initially depicted.

Active Stretch: Quadriceps, iliopsoas, rectus abdominis and transverse abdominis.

Technique:

a. Assume a kneeling position—either from Samsthiti or Bhramanasana.
b. Lift your arms and bring them to shoulder level.
c. Inhale and lift your sternum (breastbone), extending your trunk into a back extension. Point your tailbone towards your knees while moving your arms back from the sides, one by one.
d. Breathe normally and allow your ribcage to expand.
e. Continue to breathe normally and keep your neck engaged; do not drop it passively. Hold this position for 10 to 20 seconds.
f. Exit Ustrasana in the exact reverse order. You can also rest in Child's Pose for a while.

Benefits

- Opens the chest muscles

- Activates hip muscles, rear thigh muscles, back muscles, and more
- Releases tightness from the chest and shoulder muscles
- Helps improve lung capacity
- Can energise the body
- Helps alleviate back pain
- Believed to release hidden emotions from the heart

Common Mistakes to Avoid

- Steep bends from the lower back
- Moving your waist forward
- Jerky movements
- Not engaging the hip muscles

Biomechanics

The Ustrasana can be practised in closed kinetic chain (CKC) and open kinetic chain (OKC) fashions.

For a controlled descent, focus on engaging your glutes and abdominal muscles. However, this should not hinder your breathing pattern.

Ustrasana mainly activates the posterior chain of muscles, including the back, hip, and thigh muscles. Meanwhile, the pectoral muscles (pectoralis major, pectoralis minor), abdominal muscles, quadriceps, and iliopsoas stretch.

The back muscles, including the erector spinae, transversospinalis, trapezius, and latissimus dorsi, contract to create the backward extension of this asana. In OKC, the abdominal muscles contract, whereas in CKC, the rectus abdominis and transverse abdominis stretch. However, the more control you have over your abdominal muscles, the better it is for the spine.

The rhomboid muscles work in synergy with the trapezius muscles to retract and stabilise the scapulae while the pectoral muscles stretch.

The gluteal and hamstring muscles contract to extend the hips while the iliopsoas (antagonist) and quadriceps lengthen. However, avoid moving your waistline beyond your knees as it may compress the spine.

Additionally, the gluteus medius acts to rotate the legs externally, but the gluteus medius and minimus, along with the TFL, counteract this. To improve your backbend, you may use a yoga block to engage your gluteus medius, minimus, and TFL effectively.

Lastly, ensure your anterior neck muscles, the longus capitis and longus colli, remain gently active. Avoid engaging the sternocleidomastoid muscle (the largest muscle in front of the neck), as it may pull the skull towards the summit of the cervical spine (atlanto-occipital joint). Furthermore, practise the simplest version of Ustrasana in neck-related conditions—look slightly ahead and keep the chin tucked.

Modifications

- **Regression/Variation I:** To regress, place your hands by the sides of your lower back so that your thumbs are facing away from each other. This is based on the OKC movement. However, in this variation, you need to engage your abdominal muscles to sustain the movement.
- **Variation II:** Another easy variation of Ustrasana involves tucking your toes to grip the floor/mat more firmly. This helps improve balance and reduces the extent of your backbend.

- **Progression/Variation III:** If you wish to experience a deeper stretch, you can try reaching for your toes; however, this is not recommended for beginners as it may place additional strain on your facet joints.
- **Prop Work:** You can use two yoga blocks and place them outside your heels. As you bend backwards, place your hands on the blocks.

13

The Art of Rotation: Exploring Twisting Asanas

Twisting asanas focus on trunk rotation, with the twisting motion originating from the spine. Twisting is often overlooked but crucial for the thoracic spine, which has a natural affinity for it. Trunk rotation comes under the transverse plane, the most ignored plane. In this chapter, we will explore the importance of twisting asanas for our body, their biomechanical impact, and their ability to release tightness.

Vakrasana (Twisted Pose)

Etymology: *Vakra* translates to twisted; *Asana* means posture.

If you often wonder about ways to prevent lower back pain, you can do so by keeping the spine active and mobile. Various core muscles surround the spine, which work together to fortify the spine, preventing any possible damage. When we perform asanas, like the Vakrasana, our spine moves intricately. This forces the body and brain to adapt to the movement while activating several muscles.

Vakrasana is a seated spinal twist that engages our core muscles, prompting several healthcare professionals to suggest this asana as a preventive measure against lower back pain. Additionally, it can easily be practised by practitioners of all ages without any difficulty. It is also believed that Vakrasana helps stimulate our internal abdominal organs.

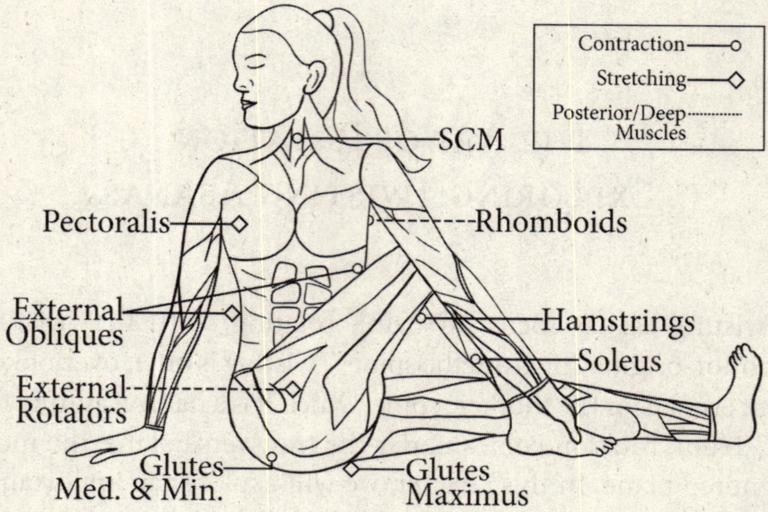

Vakrasana

Asana Category	Targeted Area	Preparatory Yogic Practices
Spinal twist	Spine (trunk rotation) (ipsilateral)	Supta Matsyendrasana (Reclining Spinal Twist Pose)
Beginner-friendly	Shoulder joints (extension)	Urdhva Mukha Pasasana (Thread the Needle Pose)
Sitting	Elbow joint (extension)	-
Asymmetrical	Hip joints (flexion)	-
Spinal therapy	Knee joint (flexion) (ipsilateral)	-
-	Knee joint (extension) (contralateral)	-

Active Stretch: Pectoralis major, glutes, and obliques.

Technique:

a. Get into Dandasana (Staff Pose), with your hands by the side of your body.
b. Bend your right knee (ipsilateral) and place the heel around your left knee (contralateral).
c. Inhale and lift your left arm (contralateral).
d. Exhale and rotate your trunk to the right. Cross your left arm to the right leg and catch hold of your right ankle if comfortable.
e. Breathe normally and keep your spine comfortably extended, while turning your neck back and rotating the trunk.
f. Hold this position for about 5 to 10 breaths. Repeat this 3 to 5 times on each side.

Benefits

- Improves spinal mobility
- Boosts spinal health
- Can aid in digestion
- Stretches and strengthens the oblique muscle
- Activates the rhomboid muscles
- Can help people with type-II diabetes and kidney-related ailments
- Improves overall posture
- Can help alleviate stress

Common Mistakes to Avoid

- Leaning onto the rear (ipsilateral) arm
- Forcing your neck into a deeper twist
- Flexing the spine
- Moving your extended leg

Biomechanics

The Vakrasana is wonderful for optimum trunk rotation. It is also quite safe for most individuals.

In several twisting yoga poses, the thoracic spine provides the most twisting movement, while the lumbar spine contributes only a small amount of trunk rotation. Additionally, the cervical spine also undergoes slight rotation.

In this asana, the rhomboid muscles are activated to retract the scapula blades, releasing the pectoralis (chest) muscles.

The sternocleidomastoid muscle (contralateral) and splenius muscles (ipsilateral) contribute to neck rotation. Similarly, the internal oblique muscle (ipsilateral) and external oblique muscle (contralateral) along with the spinal rotator muscles contribute to the entire trunk rotation.

It is worth noting that your spinal discs compress during trunk rotation. It may seem counter-intuitive because many yoga teachers advise lengthening the spine; however, this almost never occurs while rotating the trunk. To experience this, take a piece of cloth and rotate it with your arms as much as possible—you will notice your hands growing closer to each other.

Modifications

- **Regression:** If you find it difficult to catch hold of your heel/toes, it is better to cross your elbow to your bent knee.
- **Progression:** If you wish to progress into this pose, focus on rotating the upper back and moving your chest out (ipsilaterally).
- **Prop Work:** Place your rear hand on a yoga block for better grip.
- **Variation/Meru Vakrasana (Spinal Twisted Pose):** Meru Vakrasana is a progression of Vakrasana. In this variation, the bent (ipsilateral) knee is placed by crossing over the extended knee, increasing the difficulty and stretching additional muscles, such as the hip external rotators. This also activates the hip internal rotator muscles, further enhancing spinal health.

Ardha Matsyendrasana (Half Lord of the Fishes Pose)

Etymology: *Ardha* means half: *Matsya* translates to fish; Indra means the lord or king; *Asana* means posture or pose.

Ardha Matsyendrasana is a legendary pose that, according to Hatha Yoga Pradipika, can revive our digestive fire. It is an easy variation of the advanced Matsyendrasana. It is worth noting that Matsyendrasana is named after an ancient yoga guru Swami Matsyendranath of the hatha yoga tradition. He was among the biggest progenitors of hatha yoga and is revered in Buddhist and Indian traditions. Furthermore, Ardha Matsyendrasana is increasingly becoming relevant in contemporary spinal therapies.

Active Stretch: Pectoralis major, glutes, serratus anterior, and obliques.

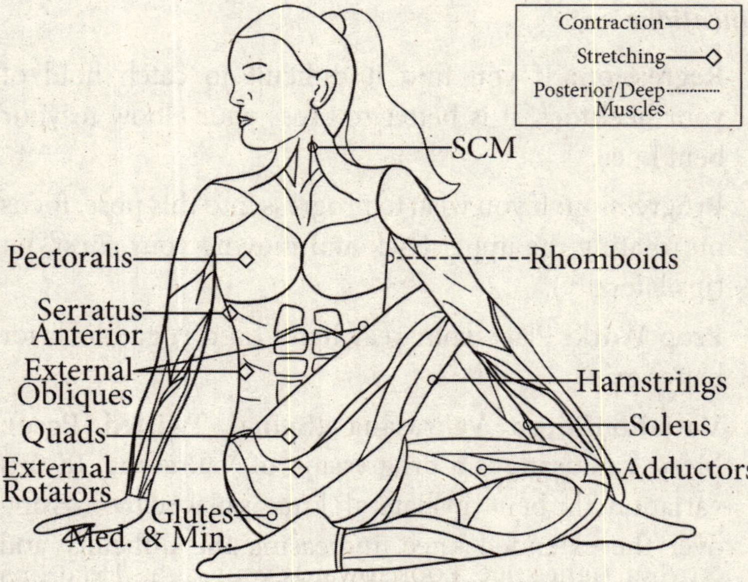

Ardha Matsyendrasana

Asana Category	Targeted Area	Preparatory Yogic Practices
Spinal twist	Spine (trunk rotation)	Vakrasana (Twisted Pose)
Beginner-friendly	Shoulder joint (flexion) (contralateral)	Ardha Padmasana (Half Lotus Pose)
Sitting	Shoulder joint (extension) (ipsilateral)	Tiryaka Tadasana (Standing Spinal Twist Pose)
Spinal therapy	Elbow joints (extension) Hip joints (flexion)	Supta Matsyendrasana (Reclining Spinal Twist Pose)
-	Knee joints (flexion)	-

Technique:

a. To practise Ardha Matsyendrasana, begin by assuming Dandasana with hands extended by your sides.
b. Bend your right leg (ipsilateral) and cross it to the left side (contralateral). Ensure your right foot's toes remain in line with the left knee.
c. Externally rotate and flex your left knee, aligning your left hip with your right hip.
d. Inhale and lift your left shoulder.
e. Exhale and rotate your trunk by focusing on your shoulders and chest.
f. Breathe normally and bend your left elbow, placing it on your right knee. Look towards your right. Hold this pose for 3 to 10 breaths.
g. Repeat the instructions in reverse to come out of this pose. Repeat it 3 to 5 times on each side.

Benefits

- Can make Paschimottanasana (Seated Forward Bend Pose) and Uttanasana (Standing Forward Bend Pose) easier
- Can help prevent backache and spinal conditions
- Stretches the often-tight hip external rotators
- Activates the vagal tone of the body
- Helps stimulate hip internal rotator muscles, which are often ignored.
- Can fuel the kidneys, liver, and pancreas (Pandey et al., 2017)
- Improves overall body posture

- Can help treat constipation and digestive conditions
- Helps release hidden stress from the upper and middle back

Common Mistakes to Avoid

- Forcing your neck into a deeper twist
- Putting all the weight on your back arm (ipsilateral) and relying on it for balance
- Excessive strain on your knees
- Flexing the spine

Biomechanics

The Ardha Matsyendrasana engages the ipsilateral internal hip rotator muscles, such as the TFL, gluteus medius, minimus, and adductor longus. It also stretches the ipsilateral external hip rotator muscles (gluteus maximus, piriformis, gemellus, and obturator internus muscles).

The hamstrings are responsible for flexing both knees, while the iliopsoas muscles flex the hip. This action releases the quadriceps muscles and contralateral glutes. Ardha Matsyendrasana is performed best when our spine is extended or neutral while twisting.

In twisting asanas, the significant twisting movement primarily comes from the thoracic spine, with some contribution from the lumbar spine, while the cervical spine also rotates—though this can be limited according to your comfort. The sternocleidomastoid muscle (contralateral) and splenius muscles (ipsilateral) contribute to neck rotation. Similarly, the contraction of the internal oblique muscle (ipsilateral) and external oblique muscle (contralateral)—along with the weak spinal rotator muscles—contributes to the entire trunk rotation. Meanwhile, antagonist muscles stretch, including the internal oblique (contralateral) and external oblique (ipsilateral).

Here, the rhomboid muscles are activated to retract the scapula blades, which stretch the pectoral muscles. Meanwhile, the serratus anterior muscles work alongside the rhomboid muscles to stabilise the movement of the scapula.

Please note that during trunk rotation, your spinal discs compress rather than lengthen.

Modifications

- **Regression:** If you find Ardha Matsyendrasana challenging, you can regress to Vakrasana (Twisted Pose).
- **Progression:** To progress, catch hold of the medial arch of the top foot (ipsilateral) and rotate your trunk further.
- **Prop Work:** To improve balance, place your rear arm on a yoga block. Keep your neck in a comfortable position, especially if you experience discomfort. Ensure that only half of your weight is distributed to your ipsilateral (rear) arm, with the rest distributed through your trunk and surrounding muscles. This will improve your balance; otherwise, you may become too dependent on your rear arm for support.

Supta Matsyendrasana (Reclining Lord of Fishes Pose)

Etymology: *Supta* means sleeping, supine, or reclining; *Matsyendra* means the Lord of Fishes or Sage Matsyendra Nath; *Asana* translates to posture.

With this simple asana, one can keep the poor everyday posture at bay. Picture yourself sitting at your desk, doing your

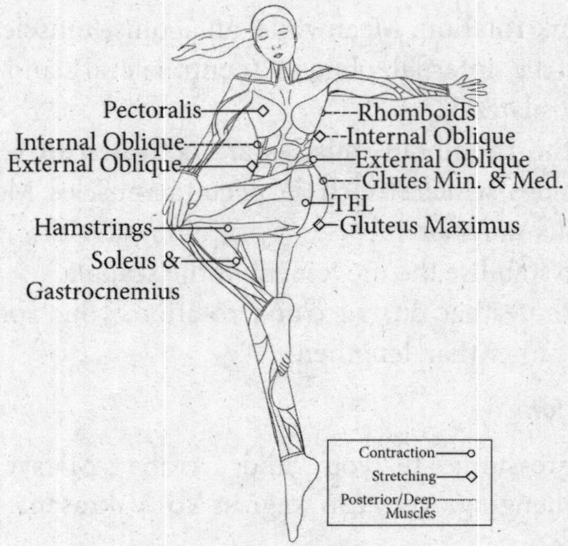

Supta Matsyendrasana

Asana Category	Targeted Area	Preparatory Yogic Practices
Twisting	Spine (rotation)	Vakrasana (Twisted Pose)
Beginner-friendly	Shoulder joint (flexion)	Kati Chakrasana (Standing Spinal Twist Pose)
Reclining/supine	Elbow joints (extension)	-
Hip-opening	Hip joint (flexion) (contralateral)	-
-	Hip joint (extension) (ipsilateral)	-
-	Knee joint (flexion) (contralateral)	-
-	Knee joint (extension) (ipsilateral)	-
-	Ankle joints (plantar flexion)	-

work diligently. However, your mind is wandering, looking for a simple solution to fix your posture, only to find the answer in a simple asana.

Supta Matsyendrasana is a gentle asana with numerous benefits. For individuals with sedentary jobs, it offers a gentle reclining spinal twist. Therefore, making it quite accommodating and effective in improving spinal health. It is believed to gently massage the internal abdominal organs, especially the gastrointestinal tract, contributing to better digestive motility.

Active Stretch: Gluteus medius and minimus (contralateral), and tensor-fascia-lata muscles.

Technique:

a. Start by assuming Shavasana (Corpse Pose) or a simple reclining position. Abduct your shoulders till your arms reach shoulder level.
b. Bend your left knee (contralateral knee and hip flexion) and gently lift the left knee at about a 90-degree angle. Slowly drop it to the right side (ipsilateral) (internal rotation of the hip).
c. Exhale and, with your right hand (ipsilateral), grab the left knee (contralateral) and then go deeper into the trunk rotation. Let your left chest expand towards the left side and your left (contralateral) thigh go towards the right side. Doing so will rotate your trunk.
d. Breathe normally and allow your body to rest in this position for about 5 to 15 breaths. If your neck allows, turn it to the opposite side.
e. Repeat it 3 to 5 times on each side.

Benefits

- Helps relieve constipation
- Can improve digestion
- Enhances spinal mobility
- Can prevent diabetes and kidney diseases
- Assists in balancing the autonomic nervous system response
- Can alleviate stress
- Helps restore energy after a hectic day
- Can help in menstruation-related issues

Common Mistakes to Avoid

- Going beyond your comfort zone
- Lifting the whole trunk

Biomechanics

While twisting, if your trunk lifts excessively, it may indicate a less mobile spine. So, in this asana, allow the primary movement to be the trunk rotation.

The trunk rotation movement originates from the coordinated action of the internal oblique muscle (ipsilateral) and the external oblique muscle (contralateral). Spinal rotators also play a minor role in trunk rotation.

The internal rotators of the hip (gluteus medius, gluteus minim-us, TFL, and adductor muscles) assist in crossing the bent leg (contralateral) towards the opposite side (ipsilateral).

This asana is comfortable for most people as the internal rotators of the hip contract while the external rotators are stretched. This creates more space for the spine, making it therapeutic for back pain in many practitioners.

Furthermore, it is essential to stabilise the scapula blades on the ground to initiate a stable trunk rotation.

Modifications

- **Regression (Prop Work):** If you wish to regress, you can add a yoga blanket or bolster, preventing you from going beyond your comfort range.
- **Progression:** If you want to progress further into the stretch, try practising with both knees bent and twisted to one side. This variation is often called Supta Matsyendrasana II. If you experience discomfort in the cervical spine (neck), keep your neck centred.

Parivrtta Utkatasana (Revolved Chair Pose)

Etymology: *Parivrtta* translates to revolved; *Utkat* means ardent; *Asana* means pose.

Parivrtta Utkatasana is a strength-oriented asana that challenges our brains and muscles, asking them to do more. It strengthens a large number of muscles in the body, especially the leg and oblique muscles. It is an intermediate yoga asana that helps burn plenty of calories. Furthermore, it involves multiple dimensions including balancing, muscle strengthening, coordination, and conditioning. Thus, the practitioner needs to have an unagitated, relaxed mind.

Active Stretch: Triceps (ipsilateral), quadriceps, erector spinae, transversospinalis, and glutes.

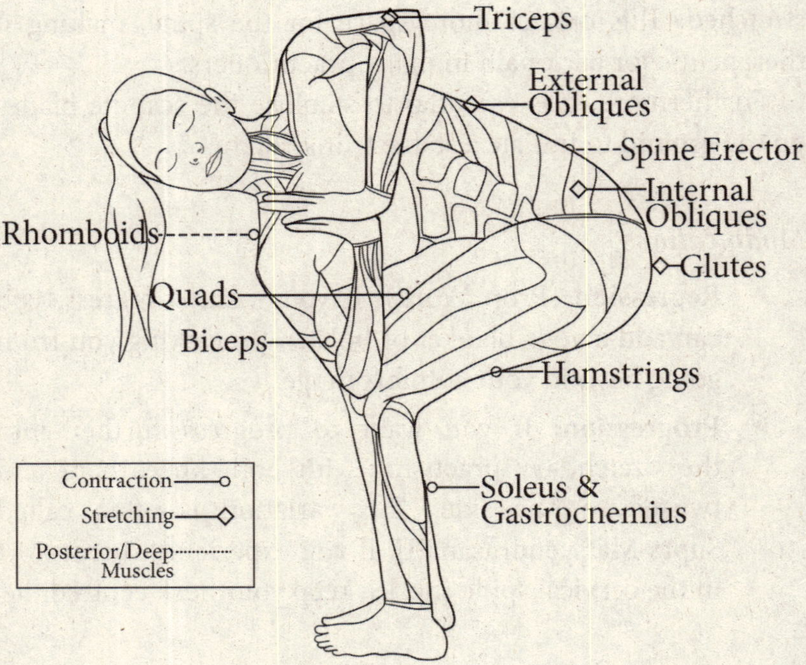

Parivrtta Utkatasana

Asana Category	Targeted Area	Preparatory Yogic Practices
Strengthening	Spine (trunk rotation, flexion) (ipsilateral)	Utkatasana (Chair Pose)
Standing	Shoulder joints (flexion)	Kati Chakrasana (Standing Spinal Twist Pose)
Trunk Rotation	Elbow joints (flexion)	-
Core	Hip joints (flexion)	-
Asymmetrical	Knee joints (flexion)	-

Technique:

a. Assume Tadasana or Samsthiti.
b. Join your palms in Namaskar or Anjali Mudra (salutation gesture).
c. Exhale and flex your knees and hip joints to get into Utkatasana (Chair Pose) with your hands in the front and legs joined together.
d. Inhale and stretch your spine up while drawing the hips out; your neck must be neutrally aligned with the spine.
e. Exhale and rotate your trunk to the right side of your body, focusing primarily on your thoracic spine (mid back). Place your left (contralateral) elbow on the outer side of the right knee (ipsilateral). Work on your core and quadriceps muscles.
f. Breathe normally and hold this position for a few breaths, about 3 to 10, and repeat it 3 to 5 times on each side.

Benefits

- Strengthens the legs, hips, core, and back
- Can prevent knee injuries
- Makes the hip joints more mobile and flexible
- Can help prevent dead butt syndrome
- Mobilises the entire trunk
- Aids in alleviating stress, anxiety, and similar conditions
- Can enhance digestion
- Helps maximise concentration
- Can help improve pancreatic and kidney health

Common Mistakes to Avoid

- Looking up
- Shifting weight to one leg
- Extensively bending the knees
- Shifting the weight on your knees and toes

Biomechanics

Parivrtta Utkatasana is one of the asanas that focuses on activating the quadriceps and gluteal muscles while they lengthen. Moreover, engaging your quadriceps and glutes is vital for protecting the knees. These muscles engage to counteract the effects of gravity, alongside the latissimus dorsi, spinal erectors, and trapezius.

It is also an asymmetrical yoga posture, meaning it should be practised on each side for an equal number of counts.

The trunk rotation movement originates from the external and internal oblique muscles, with support from the spinal rotator muscles—which are weaker. However, this motion is slightly challenging because the facet joints perform both flexion and twisting simultaneously. Therefore, I recommend engaging the core muscles to stabilise the spine.

The sternocleidomastoid muscle (contralateral) and the splenius muscles (ipsilateral) contribute to neck rotation, though the neck should always remain in a comfortable position. As with other trunk rotations, the spinal discs also experience compression. The trunk rotation should primarily originate from the spine, not from the pseudo-movement of the scapula.

The gluteal muscles are essential for stabilising the pelvis and preventing unnecessary movement. Ensure your body weight is evenly distributed across both legs, avoiding overburdening one leg while holding this pose.

Lastly, distribute your body weight evenly across all sides of your feet by engaging the toes.

Modifications

- **Regression:** If practising this pose is difficult, you can regress by assuming Utkatasana with a mild twist, instead of going all the way down.
- **Progression:** To progress in this pose, gently lift the opposite (contralateral) leg to about 90 degrees while keeping both knees intact. However, this is not recommended for intermediate or beginner practitioners.
- **Prop Work:** You can use a resistance band or yoga belt to wrap around your legs. It is advised to keep the neck aligned with the rest of the spine or move it within a comfortable range of motion.

Parivrtta Parsvakonasana (Revolved Side Angle Pose)

Etymology: *Parivrtta* means revolved; *Parsva* means side; *Kona* translates to angle; *Asana* means pose.

Trunk rotation is a movement we rarely perform in our daily routine. However, as less valuable as it may seem, trunk rotation is important for a healthy spine.

Parivrtta Parsvakonasana is a wonderful blend of concurrent balance, trunk rotation, and strengthening. During this pose, our spine undergoes intermediate rotation while the trunk is in flexion and lateral flexion. Therefore, practitioners must mindfully stabilise the body while activating the right muscles, enhancing the mind and body connection.

Active Stretch: Quadriceps, gastrocnemius, soleus, obliques, and glutes (ipsilateral).

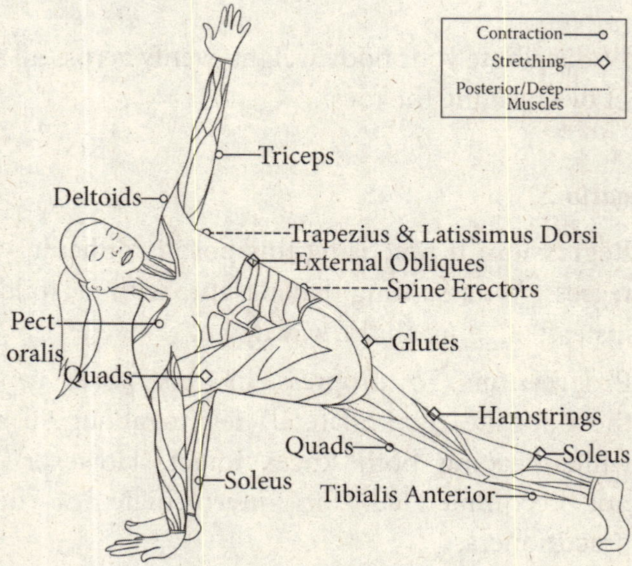

Parivrtta Parsvakonasana

Asana Category	Targeted Area	Preparatory Yogic Practices
Twisting	Spine (rotation)	Parivrtta Utkatasana (Revolved Chair Pose)
Intermediate	Shoulder joints (horizontal abduction)	Parivrtta Trikonasana (Revolved Triangle Pose)
Strengthening	Elbow joints (flexion)	Utthita Parsvakonasana (Extended Side Angle Pose)
Standing	Hip joint (flexion) (ipsilateral)	-
Hip-opening	Hip joint (extension) (contralateral)	-
-	Knee joint (flexion) (ipsilateral)	-
-	Knee joint (extension) (contralateral)	-
-	Ankle joints (dorsiflexion)	-

Technique:

a. Begin from Tadasana or Samasthiti.
b. Open your legs about four feet apart, abduct your arms at shoulder level, and bend your right knee (ipsilateral) at a 90-degree angle. Your opposite leg (contralateral) will remain extended.
c. Now, assume Anjali or Namaskar Mudra by joining your arms in the front.
d. Initiate trunk rotation towards the right and place the opposite (left) elbow (contralateral) on your right thigh (ipsilateral). Keep your neck relaxed.
e. Hold this position for about 3 to 10 breaths.
f. Repeat it 3 to 5 times on each side.

Benefits

- Can enhance digestion
- Helps overcome stress, anxiety, and depression
- Reduces the fat percentage—when combined with other strength-oriented asanas.
- Enhances concentration
- Improves the grounding through neuro-muscular coordination
- Can enhance spinal flexibility
- Trains muscles in all three planes of motion
- Strengthens the leg and trunk muscles

Common Mistakes to Avoid

- Leaning too much towards the floor
- Not regressing in experiencing vibrations

Biomechanics

This asana is a multi-dimensional exercise, meaning the movement occurs in all three planes of motion. The internal oblique muscle (ipsilateral) and external oblique muscle (contralateral), along with the spinal rotator muscles (weak), contribute to the entire trunk rotation. Similarly, the sternocleidomastoid muscle (contralateral) and splenius muscles (ipsilateral) contribute to neck rotation.

In this pose, the quadriceps muscles work to stabilise the movement, lengthening while undergoing contraction. The front quadriceps muscle (ipsilateral) stabilises, whereas the rear quadriceps muscle (contralateral) extends the knee.

Similarly, ipsilateral hip flexion is initiated by the iliopsoas (agonist), the front glutes (antagonist) contract while lengthening to stabilise, and the rear glutes contract to extend the hip against gravity.

When we perform the Namaskar Mudra, it activates the pectoralis (chest) muscles.

The latissimus dorsi, rhomboids, quadratus lumborum, transversospinalis, and transverse abdominis stabilise the trunk.

Dorsiflexion in the rear leg activates the contralateral tibialis anterior muscle and stretches the soleus and gastrocnemius. In the front leg, activating the toes engages the soleus and gastrocnemius.

Modifications

- **Regression/Variation I (Preparatory Adaptations):** To regress in this pose, gently drop your opposite knee down (contralateral). Doing so will help stabilise the body and reduce the stress on your quadriceps muscles.

- **Progression (Original Asana):** To progress in this asana, try placing your opposite arm down (contralateral) and raising the same-side arm (ipsilateral) towards the ceiling.
- **Prop Work:** If you wish to attempt the full version but cannot reach the floor, use a yoga block.
- **Variation II:** You can also clench your hands while performing this asana, creating a deeper trunk rotation.
- **Variation III (Prop Work):** Using a yoga chair, you can place your same-side thigh (ipsilateral) on it, making the asana easier to perform.

14
The Power of Lateral Bending Asanas

Lateral bending asanas, also called side bends, are practised in the frontal plane. They play a vital role in keeping the spine healthy while stretching some muscles that are otherwise barely used. Side bends can ease our respiratory system, in turn releasing hidden tensions. They also release stiffness from the neck, ribs, spine, shoulders, and legs. Whether incorporated into a larger yoga sequence or practised on their own, lateral bending asanas are a powerful way to unlock physical tension and increase body awareness.

Tiryaka Tadasana (Swaying Palm Tree Pose)

Etymology: *Tiryaka* means swaying, sideward, transverse, or lateral; *Tada* translates to palm tree; *Asana* means posture.

The lateral bends create an effective synergy between the internal and external intercostal muscles, the accessory muscles of respiration, by isolating and lengthening them simultaneously. Does this create a disjunction between the two sides of the intercostal muscles? Yes, we seldom realise that we tend to lean towards one side of the body. Over time, this repetitive pattern causes one side to become tighter than the other. Tiryaka Tadasana can help overcome this imbalance and promote more effective respiration.

Active Stretch: Obliques, quadratus lumborum (contralateral), SCM, scalene, and splenius.

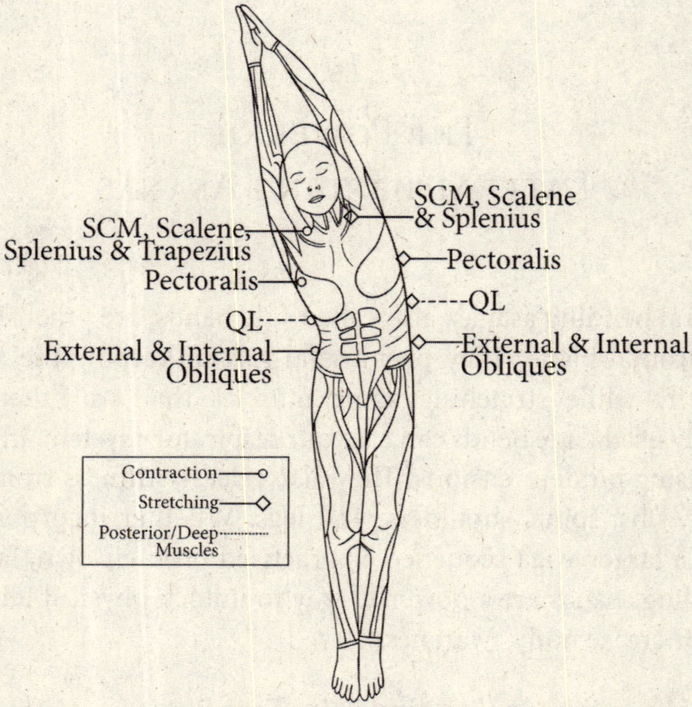

Tiryaka Tadasana

Asana Category	Targeted Area	Preparatory Yogic Practices
Side/lateral bend	Spine (lateral flexion)	Samasthiti (Equal Standing Pose)
Beginner-friendly	Shoulder joints (abduction)	Tadasana (Palm Tree Pose)
Standing	Hip joints (adduction)	Parsva Sukhasana (Easy Pose with Side Bend)
-	Knee joints (extension)	-
-	Ankle joints (neutral)	-

Technique:

a. Assume Tadasana or Samasthiti and place your legs about hip-width apart.
b. Ensure your body weight is evenly distributed.
c. Inhale and stretch your arms over your head, palms facing each other (internal rotation of the shoulders).
d. Exhale and laterally bend your body to the right side, up to a comfortable range (about 30–45 degrees).
e. Breathe normally and hold this position for about 5 to 10 breaths.
f. Gently come back to Samasthiti.
g. Repeat 3 to 5 times on each side.

Benefits

- Works on our oblique and spine rotator muscles
- Mobilises the spinal joints
- Can stimulate various internal abdominal organs like the liver, pancreas, and kidneys
- Releases external and internal intercostal muscles
- Can relieve type 2 diabetes
- Can prevent kidney and gallbladder stones
- Improves overall spatial awareness of the body

Common Mistakes to Avoid

- Excessive lateral bending
- External rotation of the hips
- Bending forward while bending laterally
- Straining your neck
- Extreme lateral bending if you have sciatica

Biomechanics

In Tiryaka Tadasana, facet joints contribute to lateral flexion. Here, the motion is based on the frontal plane.

Ensure you distribute your weight equally on both legs as it activates peroneal muscles in the ipsilateral leg while stretching the other.

Tiryaka Tadasana is a pose that requires a larger base of support. This is because a smaller base of support reduces lateral flexion of the trunk and stability.

To keep your neck comfortable, you can maintain retracted and downward shoulder blades, providing more room for the cervical spine.

To prevent any injury, engage the core muscles effectively, as doing so initiates the movements efficiently, stabilising the entire spine.

Modifications

- **Regression:** To ease into this asana, only bend laterally to a comfortable level. Gradually progress from there.
- **Progression:** If you want to advance to Tiryaka Tadasana, try the Trikonasana (Triangle Pose) with the open kinetic chain variation.
- **Prop Work:** You can use a resistance band or yoga belt to wrap around your legs.

Utthita Trikonasana (Extended Triangle Pose)

Etymology: *Utthita* translates to extended; *Trikon* means triangle; *Asana* means pose.

Named after a series of triangles that it forms, Utthita Trikonasana works on various aspects of the body including stretching, balancing, strengthening, and mobilising.

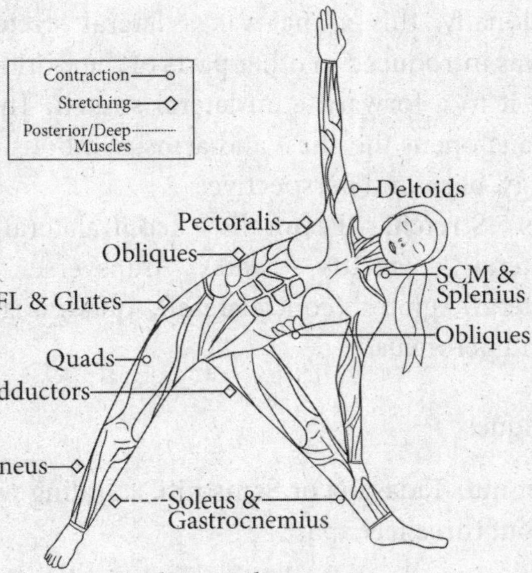

Utthita Trikonasana

Asana Category	Targeted Area	Preparatory Yogic Practices
Beginner-friendly	Spine (lateral flexion)	Virabhadrasana-II (Warrior-II Pose)
Lateral bending	Shoulder joints (abduction)	Tiryaka Tadasana (Swaying Palm Tree Pose)
Standing	Elbow joints (extension)	Alternate Toe Touch (practice)
Balancing	Hip joint (flexion) (external rotation) (ipsilateral)	-
Chest/heart opening	Hip joint (flexion) (internal rotation) (contralateral)	-
-	Knee joints (extension)	-
-	Ankle joints (plantar flexion)	-

Traditionally, this asana was a lateral stretch; however, when it was introduced in other parts of the world, some gurus modified it to a forward cum lateral stretch. The traditional Trikonasana opens the chest and arms, symbolising accepting new energy, bliss, and perspective.

Active Stretch: Pectoralis (contralateral), obliques (contralateral), rectus and transverse abdominis (contralateral), glutes (contralateral), quadratus lumborum, biceps, and peroneus.

Technique:

a. Get into Tadasana or Samsthiti, standing with your feet about three feet apart.

b. Place your heels and toes on the sides of a rectangle, parallel to each other.

c. Contract your quadriceps—doing so may pull your knee plates up. Go for an axial extension of the spine while keeping the pelvis neutral.

d. Maintaining the neutral position of the pelvis, gently turn your right toe outwards (external rotation of the hip) at a 90-degree angle.

e. Similarly, slightly turn your left leg inwards towards your right leg (left hip internal rotation). Ensure both heels are aligned.

f. Firmly grip the floor with your toes to ensure better engagement of the calf muscle and for stability.

g. Micro-bend your knees, especially the right knee.

h. Inhale and lift your arms to shoulder level.

i. Exhale and bend laterally to your right (ipsilateral) and ensure a gradual curvature of your spine. Allow your pelvis to move only at a later stage, to be in sync with the spine.

j. Place your right hand on your shin, ankle, or a yoga block for support.
k. Your arms should ideally be aligned, with the left arm perpendicular to the floor.
l. Traditionally, it is advised to gaze at your superior thumb if comfortable. However, it is better to keep the neck facing the front (anterior) side of the body to avoid strain from gravity.
m. Breathe normally and hold this asana for 5 to 10 breaths or as per your capacity. Mindfully observe your body, stretches, and contractions.
n. Smoothly ease back by following the instructions in reverse. Repeat this 3 to 5 times on each side.

Benefits

- Stretches the inner thigh muscles
- Activates and stretches oblique muscles
- Can stimulate intra-abdominal soft muscles
- Believed to improve abdominal and renal functions
- Enhances bone density
- Prevents hip joint osteoarthritis
- Calms the mind by releasing tight muscles
- Improves equilibrioception or sense of balance
- Tones the external rotators of the hips.
- Can help prepare us for meditative Asanas.

Common Mistakes to Avoid

- Slouching while bending laterally
- Turning your chest towards the floor
- Jerky movements
- Hyperextending the knees
- Moving your pelvis in the initial stage
- Placing your hand on the knee

Biomechanics

Beginners should ensure they do not hyperextend their ipsilateral knee. To avoid this, keep a slight bend in the knees.

The cervical spine is an integral part of the rest of the spine. Therefore, it is crucial to keep it aligned with the rest of the spine. Unless you intend to practise the full form of Triangle Pose, keep your head comfortably facing forward.

As mentioned earlier, some practitioners tend to tilt their chest towards the floor, which causes this asana to become a forward bend rather than a lateral one. I suggest focusing on a lateral bend, as lateral stretches are often neglected in our everyday lives. Moreover, they are essential to maintain holistic health.

Asymmetry between the two sides of the body is common, and Triangle Pose can help minimise it. It is one of the asymmetrical asanas that isolates and stretches the tighter muscles on each side, helping the body achieve equilibrium.

Additionally, in this asana, several muscles on the ipsilateral side contract, including the external and internal obliques, rectus and transverse abdominis, quadratus lumborum, and erector spinae muscles. Meanwhile, muscles on the contralateral side release, including the contralateral external and internal obliques, rectus and transverse abdominis, quadratus lumborum, and erector spinae muscles.

In the ipsilateral leg, primarily the adductor, hamstring, and tibialis anterior muscles are stretched upon contracting the quadriceps, soleus, and gastrocnemius muscles. On the other hand, in the contralateral leg, the hamstring, peroneus, soleus, and gastrocnemius muscles are stretched while contracting the quadriceps and tibialis anterior muscles.

This asana brings most of the body into a closed kinetic chain movement, except for the upper arm. For better alignment, avoid shifting your pelvis to the opposite side; let the movement naturally synchronise with lateral trunk flexion.

Pelvic rotation may occur if your adductors are shortened, and your spine may rotate to compensate. I suggest allowing some hip rotation while minimising pelvic rotation. If you experience slight pain in the front knee, it may indicate a lack of hip mobility.

Senior yoga practitioners may encounter issues with instability. In such cases, I suggest widening the base of support. This can be achieved by increasing the gap between the legs or turning the rear foot slightly outward.

Modifications

- **Regression:** If you have spinal, pelvic, or hip joint issues, you may slightly ease into the lateral bend, as you are likely to have tight hip and hamstring muscles. Hence, the pelvis needs to be relaxed.
- **Progression:** To progress, gently release support from your lower hand and align both arms. This brings your upper body into an open kinetic chain movement, resulting in more stretches.
- **Prop Work:** You can use a yoga block if you cannot reach forward. Additionally, the yoga block helps remove the excess load from your knees. Try placing it behind your

lower leg. Lastly, in case you experience any discomfort in your neck, maintain a comfortable position.

Utthita Parsvakonasana (Extended Side Angle Pose)

Etymology: *Utthita* means extended or lifted; *Parsva* translates to side or lateral; *Kona* means angle; *Asana* means posture.

In Utthita Parsvakonasana, one side of the body forms an angle with the floor, which gives the pose its name. This powerful asana—when performed with the correct alignment, flow, and breathing technique—burns calories. If you want to strengthen your core, include Utthita Parsvakonasana in your yoga sequence.

Active Stretch: Quadriceps (ipsilateral), obliques (contralateral), peroneus, and glutes.

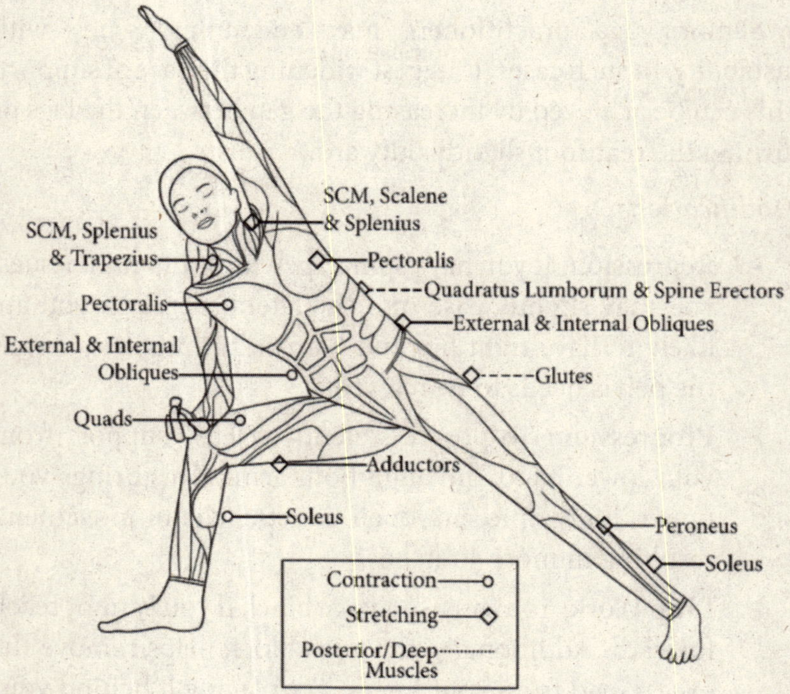

Utthita Parsvakonasana

Asana Category	Targeted Area	Preparatory Yogic Practices
Side/lateral bend	Spine (lateral flexion)	Trikonasana (Triangle Pose)
Beginner-friendly	Shoulder joints (abduction)	Tiryaka Tadasana (Swaying Palm Tree Pose)
Standing	Hip joint (abduction) (external rotation)	Parsva Sukhasana (Easy Pose with Side Bend)
Hip-opening	Hip joint (abduction) (internal rotation)	-
-	Knee joint (flexion) (ipsilateral)	-
-	Knee joint (extension) (contralateral)	-
-	Ankle joints (dorsiflexion)	-

Technique:

a. Begin with Samasthiti.

b. Stand with your feet about four feet apart. Move your right foot's toes towards your right side (ipsilateral). Raise your arms till they reach your shoulders.

c. Bend your right knee (ipsilateral) at about a 90-degree angle.

d. For an easy variation, exhale and bend laterally to the side from your waist. Rest your right forearm (ipsilateral) on your right knee (ipsilateral). Raise your left arm (contralateral) further and align it with the rest of your body, palm facing downwards.

e. In the actual variation, place your right palm (ipsilateral) on the mat in front of your right foot (ipsilateral). By doing so, your right palm and right heel (ipsilateral) should be aligned with the left foot's toes (contralateral).
f. Breathe normally and hold this position for about 3 to 10 breaths.
g. After completing one round, follow the instructions in reverse to come back.
h. Repeat it 3 to 5 times on each side.

Benefits

- Strengthens the entire body
- Activates the obliques, quadriceps, and other leg muscles
- Stretches the legs and obliques
- Helps reduce fat from the body, especially when practised sequentially with other strength-based asanas
- Releases external and internal intercostal muscles
- Enhances body awareness
- Supports the arch of the feet
- Builds physical endurance

Common Mistakes to Avoid

- Lifting your head or turning it
- Bending forward or sideward
- Too much or too little gap between the legs

Biomechanics

Utthita Parsvakonasana may seem similar to Virabhadrasana II (Warrior II) in some aspects; however, here, the leg muscles work more intensively to stabilise and counterbalance the weight of the trunk. Additionally, it involves more closed kinetic chain motion properties than Virabhadrasana II.

Keep your neck stable and avoid tilting it upwards to prevent discomfort.

Some practitioners tend to tilt their chest towards the floor, which causes this asana to become a forward bend rather than a lateral one. I recommend avoiding this.

The asymmetrical nature of the pose helps bring equilibrium to the body while activating and stretching specific muscles in isolation. However, do not be overly concerned with asymmetry, as a certain degree of it is perfectly natural.

Ensure that you grip the ground with your toes and fingers, as this activates additional muscles that help alleviate tension on your joints.

In this pose, the femur bone rolls over the tibial shaft to create a 90-degree angle, making strong activation of the ipsilateral quadriceps and hamstrings essential.

Parsvakonasana is a complex movement that involves rigorous and simultaneous activation of the core, spinal erectors, latissimus dorsi, rhomboids, trapezius, and deltoid muscles. It primarily releases the contralateral adductors, external hip rotators, and iliopsoas.

If you are practising the palm-touch variation of Parsvakonasana, avoid placing too much weight on your ipsilateral arm. Instead, put 50 per cent or more of the weight on your leg muscles and the rest on your arm.

Modifications

- **Regression:** If you find the contractions too intense—especially in the quads—you can opt for an easier variation of the Parsvakonasana, where you should reduce the distance between your feet and place your same side arm (ipsilateral) on your knee. Keep in mind that this variation may compromise stability as it narrows the base of support.
- **Progression:** To progress in this pose, you can try the arm-clenched variation of Baddha Parsvakonasana (Bound Side Angle Pose). Here, your ipsilateral hand is held by the contralateral hand, which adds extra load to the ipsilateral quadriceps muscles.
- **Prop Work:** If you're unable to place your palm on the floor, you can use a yoga block for support.
- **Modification:** For those with cervical spine (neck) conditions, it's recommended to keep your gaze forward.

Parivrtta Janu Sirsasana (Revolved Head-to-Knee Pose)

Etymology: Parivrtta translates to revolved: *Janu* means thigh; *Sirsa* is head; *Asana* means posture.

The effects of stress, anxiety, and depression are reflected in our muscles as well. Often, under stress, some of our muscles tense up even when unengaged, like the pelvic floor muscles, which are often overactive and can lead to various issues such as constipation, other digestive disorders, and dissatisfaction. One can overcome these issues by practising Parivrtta Janu Sirsasana, as it helps ease the mind and body, enhancing overall health.

Active Stretch: Core (contralateral), erector spinae (contralateral), iliopsoas (contralateral), glutes, and triceps.

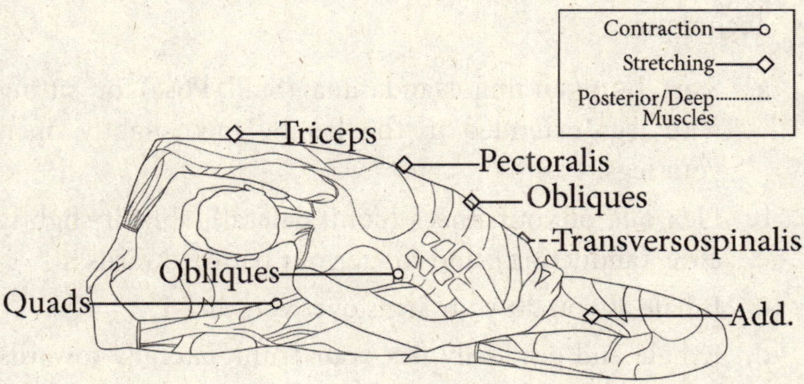

Parivrtta Janu Sirsasana

Asana Category	Targeted Area	Preparatory Yogic Practices
Sitting	Spine (lateral flexion) (rotation)	Janu Sirsasana (Head-to-Knee Pose)
Twisting	Shoulder joints (flexion)	Baddha Konasana (Bound Angle Pose)
Lateral Bend	Elbow joints (flexion)	-
Intermediate	Hip joints (flexion) (abduction)	-
-	Knee joint (extension) (ipsilateral)	-
-	Knee joint (flexion) (contralateral)	-
-	Ankle joint (dorsiflexion) (ipsilateral)	-
-	Ankle joint (plantar flexion) (contralateral)	-

Technique:

a. Start by assuming Dandasana (Staff Pose) or sitting with legs extended in the front. Now, slightly open your legs.
b. Flex one of your knees (contralateral), shift it slightly away (abduction), and rotate your trunk towards it.
c. Inhale as you lift your arms over your head.
d. Exhale and gradually flex your trunk laterally towards your extended knee.
e. Breathe normally and hold this position for 3 to 10 breaths.
f. Repeat the instructions to come back to the starting position. Practise this sequence 3 to 5 times on each side.

Benefits

- Believed to stimulate the liver, kidneys, and pancreas
- Can improve digestion
- Stretches the rear thigh, back, and inner thigh muscles
- Opens the chest and side muscles
- Can mobilise the spine
- Can cure insomnia
- Can lift your mood

Common Mistakes to Avoid

- Bending your neck too much.
- Getting into this asana forcefully
- Steep bending
- Excessive lateral flexion

Biomechanics

Aim for a gradual side bend rather than a steep one. While practising Parivrtta Janu Sirsasana, your spinal (intervertebral) discs move to the opposite side. The facet joints compress on the bending side while gliding against each other. Meanwhile, on the non-bending side, the facet joints open a minute cavity.

If you perform a steep lateral bend in Parivrtta Janu Sirsasana, it places your spinal discs in an uncomfortable position due to deep compression. Therefore, engage your muscles as much as possible and avoid practising this asana without proper muscle engagement.

The side bending comes from the ipsilateral muscles, including the iliopsoas, external and internal obliques, rectus and transverse abdominis, erector spinae, latissimus dorsi, and trapezius.

Trunk rotation is achieved by the contralateral external oblique and the ipsilateral internal oblique muscles.

You will typically experience a stretch on the contralateral latissimus dorsi, trapezius, iliopsoas, internal oblique, rectus and transverse abdominis, and erector spinae muscles.

The quadratus lumborum muscle on the ipsilateral side contracts to contribute to movement and stabilise the pelvis, while the quadratus lumborum on the contralateral side stretches.

Additionally, the biceps and deltoid muscles assist in holding the foot.

Parivrtta Janu Sirsasana also stretches the ipsilateral glutes, hamstring, adductor, gastrocnemius, and soleus muscles.

On the contralateral side, the adductor, sartorius, and quadriceps muscles bend the knee, while the contralateral gluteal muscles abduct the hip joint and stabilise the pelvis to support the movement.

Modifications

- **Regression:** You can regress by bending only slightly and keeping your arms parallel.
- **Progression:** To progress into this pose, focus on engaging multiple muscles without interrupting your breath.
- **Prop Work:** You can also use a yoga strap or belt and place it on the medial side of your ipsilateral foot. This will help pull your body gradually.
- **Yin Yoga:** Place a yoga bolster on the turning side to limit motion and feel mild stretches.

Vasisthasana (Side Plank Pose)

Etymology: *Vasistha* is the legendary Sage Vasistha; *Asana* means pose.

Vasisthasana is the epitome of body and mind connection. Vasisthasana is named after the legendary Sage Vasistha. It is an intense pose that requires intricate muscle contractions. In this asana, the body is subject to gravity in a unique manner, involving invaluable inputs from our senses. Additionally, it is also ideal for people aiming for a lean body.

Active Stretch: Obliques (contralateral), TFL and glutes (contralateral), peroneus, and sternocleidomastoid (contralateral).

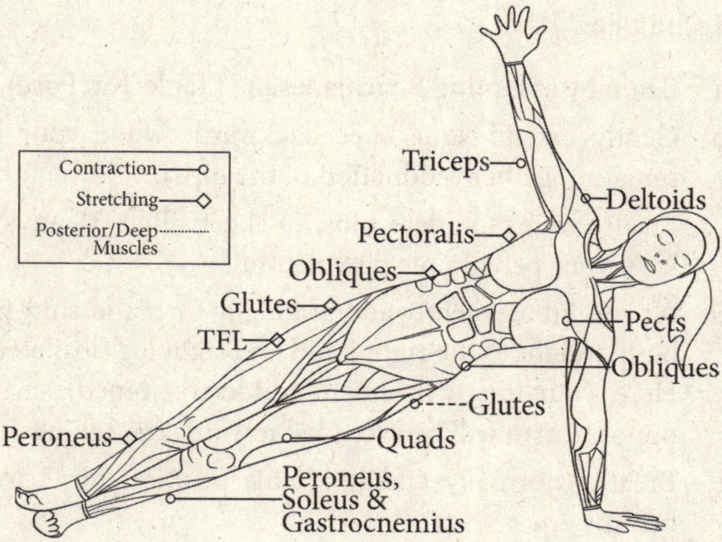

Vasisthasana

Asana Category	Targeted Area	Preparatory Yogic Practices
Lateral bend	Spine (lateral flexion)	Tiryaka Tadasana (Swaying Palm Tree Pose)
Intermediate	Shoulder joints (abduction)	Makara Adho Mukha Svanasana (Dolphin Plank Pose)
Strengthening	Elbow joints (extension)	Phalakasana (Plank Pose)
Balancing	Pelvis (neutral)	-
-	Hip joints (extension)	-
-	Knee joints (extension)	-
-	Ankle joints (dorsiflexion)	-

Technique:

a. Begin by assuming Bharmanasana (Table Top Pose).
b. Gently extend your knee backwards while your legs remain together (adduction of the hips).
c. Ensure your shoulders, hips, and heels align. Meanwhile, keep your pelvis and spine neutral.
d. As you inhale, gently and gradually turn and shift your body weight to the right hand and right leg (ipsilateral). Here, your legs will remain adducted (joined) and the opposite arm will be extended towards the ceiling.
e. Breathe normally and hold this position for 3 to 10 breaths.
f. Return to the starting position by gradually lowering your body. Repeat this 3 to 5 times on each side.

Benefits

- Strengthens the core, chest, and shoulder muscles
- Improves the sense of balance
- Helps improve focus
- Enhances the neuromuscular coordination
- Can help shred body fat
- Boosts the resting metabolic rate.

Common Mistakes to Avoid

- Not mobilising and warming up the joints
- Lifting the waist too much
- Lowering the waist
- Wobbling

Biomechanics

Lifting the waist too high may place additional strain on your muscles, and compensation could lead to stress on other muscles and joints.

Ensure a firm grip of your toes and fingers on the mat to activate the digitorum muscles.

This asana requires the co-contraction of various opposing muscles, engaging most of the body's major muscles.

Keep a slight bend in your elbows to activate the triceps and forearm muscles more effectively, reducing the load on the soft tissues of the elbows.

The quadriceps and glutes work together to stabilise the pelvis. The natural tendency in this asana is to fall due to gravity; therefore, the upper ipsilateral external and internal oblique muscles undergo deeper contraction than the lower contralateral external and internal obliques.

In Vasisthasana, the quadratus lumborum, spinal erectors, trapezius, and latissimus dorsi play a crucial role in stabilising the pelvis.

To maintain stability and protect the shoulder joints, the deltoids, triceps, and rotator cuff muscles must engage together. Additionally, the scapulae should rest against the ribcage, facilitating better activation of the serratus anterior and trapezius muscles.

Modifications

- **Regression (Easy Modification):** If the standard variation of the Vasisthasana is too challenging, place the toes of both feet on the ground, aligning them with each other to increase stability and support.
- **Regression (Variation I):** To make the pose easier and more stable, you can bend the lower elbow and rest

your entire forearm on the floor. This increases the base of support.

- **Progression:** To progress, try lifting the top leg slightly higher to activate more muscles.
- **Prop Work:** Use a towel or blanket to support your forearm in the forearm variation.
- **Wall Support:** If you have trouble with balance, you can use a wall for support to enhance the overall stability of the pose.

Lastly, remember to mobilise your joints adequately before or after practising Vasisthasana.

15

The Mind-Body Connection: Stress Release through Hip-Opening Asanas

Hip-opening asanas target the stiff hip muscles. Multiple muscles are located in and around the pelvic girdle, which can become stiff due to prolonged sitting, standing, a sedentary lifestyle, or other daily activities. We often fail to realise that stress directly affects the pelvic floor muscles, which are vital for our excretory functions and can lead to emotional and social discomfort. In this chapter, we will explore the benefits and biomechanics of hip-opening asanas.

Malasana (Deep Squat Pose)

Etymology: *Mal* translates to excretion; *Asana* means pose or posture.

Historically, Malasana was popular among Indians as well as other Asian traditions. In fact, it still is. It is also often wrongly translated as the 'Garland Pose'.

Its popularity is attributed to its ability to keep the hips, knees, and ankle joints mobile. Additionally, from a health standpoint, it offers us a great lifestyle, phenomenal digestion, and beyond. Malasana helps improve digestive health by enhancing blood circulation to the stomach and reducing the blood supply to the legs. This contributes to improved functioning of the internal organs.

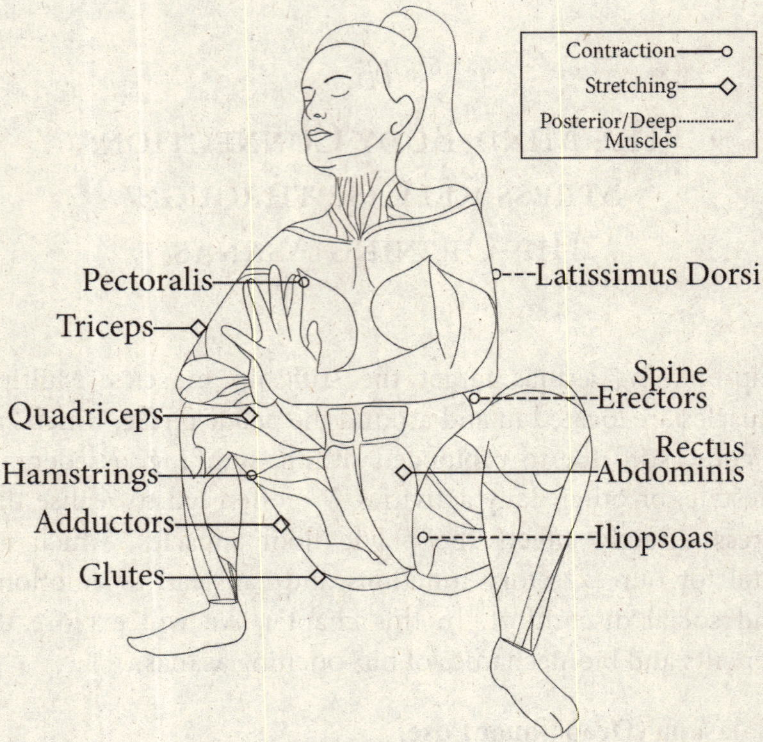

Malasana

Asana Category	Targeted Area	Preparatory Yogic Practices
Hip-opening	Spine (extension)	Utthan Pristhasana (Lizard Pose)
Sitting asana	Shoulder joints (flexion)	Agnistambhasana (Firelog Pose)
Beginner-friendly	Elbow joints (flexion)	Baddha Konasana (Bound Angle Pose)
-	Hip joints (flexion)	-
-	Knee joints (flexion)	-
-	Ankle joints (dorsiflexion)	-

Active Stretch: Glutes, soleus, and gastrocnemius.

Technique:

a. Begin by getting into Samasthiti (Equal Standing Pose). Draw your legs shoulder-width apart and assume Anjali or Namaskar Mudra with your fingers.
b. Exhale and gently bend your knees and hip joints simultaneously to their maximum extent. Allow your knees to go beyond your ankles, as this will provide them enough room to bend.
c. Inhale and move your toes outwards, by externally rotating your hips, at a maximum of a 45-degree angle. Push the inner side of your knees with your elbows—this will stretch the adductor muscles.
d. Breathe normally and draw your hips back, lengthening your entire spine including your neck.
e. Hold this position for 3 to 10 breaths, depending on your comfort.
f. Take deep breaths and come back to your original position slowly and gently.

Benefits

- Stretches the gluteal, adductor, and quadriceps muscles
- Can help prepare for child delivery (prenatal yoga)
- Helps mobilise the entire hip joint
- Strengthens the pelvic floor muscles
- Improves digestion
- Can improve fertility

Common Mistakes to Avoid

- Imbalances
- Drawing legs too wide or too close
- Rounding the back
- Jutting the neck forward
- Dropping your hips to the floor
- Jerky movements

Biomechanics

In Malasana, several leg and core muscles work together to prevent the body from losing balance. People often lose balance for various reasons. One reason is limited dorsiflexion caused by tight soleus, gastrocnemius, and tibialis posterior muscles, and sometimes due to less mobile ankle joints. Tight hip muscles can also contribute to a limited range of motion of the hip joints, leading to imbalance. Additionally, structural variations and tight spine erector muscles, induced by improper everyday posture, can also limit the ability to perform Malasana.

In Malasana, the hip abductor muscles (gluteus minimus and medius) initiate the abduction, while the hip external rotators initiate external rotation of the hips, contributing to adductor muscle stretch. When moving from Samasthiti to deep squat, ensure that you allow your knees to go slightly ahead and outwards, allowing the ankle joints to bend (dorsiflex) more naturally following the right centre of gravity pattern.

Kinesiology: Practising malasana helps improve digestion and reproductive health. Performing Malasana also redirects blood circulation and attention to the abdominal and pelvic area, thus benefiting the reproductive and digestive systems.

Modifications

- **Regression:** To simplify, you can practise it with a wall support.
- **Progression:** To advance, you can try Kagasana (Raven Pose), where you join the legs in Malasana while keeping the feet neutral and parallel.
- **Yoga Props:** Use a yoga block or blanket if you find it difficult to hold this asana.

Sucirandhrasana (Eye of the Needle Pose)

Etymology: *Suci* means needle; *Randhra* translates to hole; *Asana* means pose.

Sucirandhrasana has a deep therapeutic application and is often advised by orthopaedists, physiotherapists, and yoga teachers to recover from spinal injuries. The exact reason for this lies in the deep hip compartment. Our external leg rotators (piriformis, gemellus, obturator internus, etc.) are often tight due to our walking and sleeping patterns. This asana stretches these deep gluteal muscles, resulting in a stable pelvis. A stable pelvis enables freer spinal movements.

Also, besides 'Eye of the Needle', the name Supta Kapotasana or Reclining Pigeon Pose is commonly used. However, the name Supta Kapotasana could be misleading as it resembles the forward-bending variation of the Kapotasana (Pigeon Pose).

Active Stretch: Glutes, quadriceps, and hip external rotators.

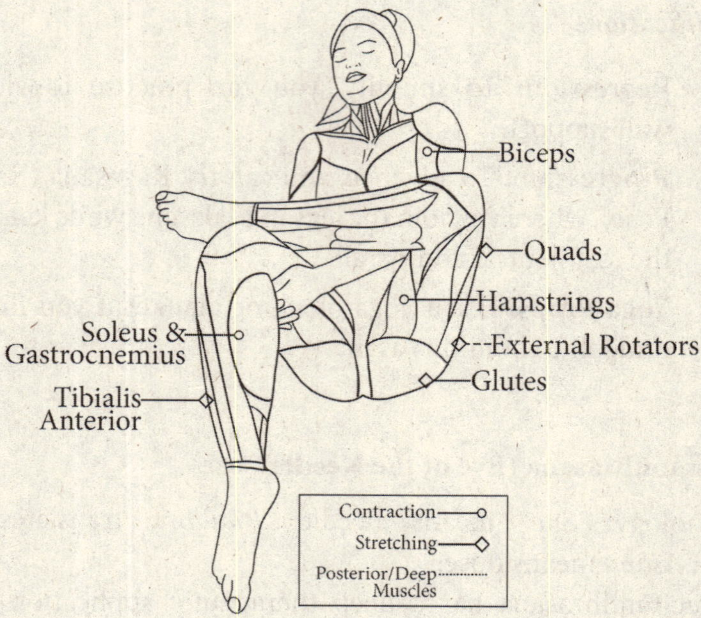

Sucirandhrasana

Asana Category	Targeted Area	Preparatory Yogic Practices
Hip-opening	Spine (slight flexion)	Kapotasana (Pigeon Pose)
Reclining/supine	Shoulder joints (flexion)	Wind Releasing Pose (Pawan Muktasana)
Beginner-friendly	Elbow joints (extension)	-
-	Pelvis (posterior pelvic tilt)	-
-	Hip joints (flexion) (ipsilateral external rotation)	-
-	Knee joints (flexion)	-
-	Ankle joints (dorsiflexion)	-

Technique:

a. Recline in Shavasana or a simple supine position.
b. Have a hip-width gap between your legs. Flex your knees and place your heels close to the hip joints.
c. Slowly externally rotate the right leg (ipsilateral) and place the right ankle slightly below the left knee (contralateral).
d. Exhale and, with your hands, grab your contralateral leg's thigh, pulling it towards your upper body. Allow your legs to lift.
e. Inhale and move your right knee away from your upper body.
f. Breathe normally and hold this position for 5 to 10 breaths.
g. Repeat 3 to 5 times on each side.

Benefits

- Helps overcome deep gluteal syndrome
- Stretches hip muscles
- Helps mobilise the hip joints
- Can improve digestion
- Therapeutic for various spinal ailments
- Helps ease the pelvic floor muscles
- Can help ease the mind

Common Mistakes to Avoid

- Extending the opposite leg
- Lifting your chest off the floor
- Moving your chin up

Biomechanics

The sciatic nerve, which passes through the sciatic notch, is often compressed by the surrounding muscles—primarily, the hip external rotator muscles (piriformis, gemellus, and obturator internus muscles). However, sometimes the hamstring muscles can also compress the sciatic nerve. Sciatic impingements of non-discogenic origin are called deep gluteal syndrome. The Sucirandhrasana helps overcome several of these compressions; hence, medical professionals often suggest practising it, especially for lower-back pain.

The hip external rotators, piriformis, gemellus, and obturator internus muscles, externally rotate the ipsilateral leg. However, in the final Sucirandhrasana, these muscles are lengthened while they stretch.

The ipsilateral sartorius muscle helps to externally rotate the hip and bend the knee, while the hamstring muscles flex the knees. In the contralateral leg, the quadriceps muscles may also act to prevent gravitational pull.

The iliopsoas muscles help in flexing the hip, enabling us to lift the legs. While assuming this asana, gluteal muscles stretch as they stabilise the pelvis.

Our spinal muscles, including erector spinae, transversospinalis, and quadratus lumborum are also mildly stretched.

Lastly, the tibialis anterior and peroneal muscles (longus and brevis) contribute to ankle stability.

Modifications

- **Regression (Modification):** If you cannot practise this asana due to any limitation, mimic the essence of the pose while sitting on a chair.

- **Progression:** You can aim to bring your legs further up.
- **Prop Work:** You can also use a yoga strap or belt to hold your thighs if you are unable to do so.

Utthan Pristhasana (Lizard Pose)

Etymology: *Utthan* means stretch or release, *Pristha* translates to page; *Asana* means posture.

If you are looking for an asana that obliterates fatigue from the body after a long day at work, Lizard Pose is your answer! Utthan Pristhasana is among the yoga postures that specifically focus on the hip muscles—it is an intense hip muscle stretch that also engages several upper body muscles including the shoulders, biceps, triceps, and chest. A hip-opening session is certainly incomplete without the Lizard Pose.

Active Stretch: Latissimus dorsi, spine erectors, quads, and glutes.

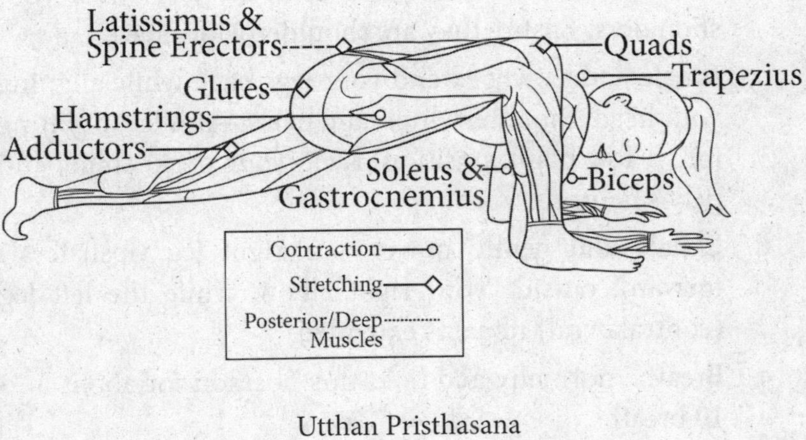

Utthan Pristhasana

Asana Category	Targeted Area	Preparatory Yogic Practices
Hip opening	Shoulder joints (flexion)	Makara Adho Mukha Svanasana (Dolphin Plank Pose)
Intermediate	Elbow joints (flexion)	Phalakasana (Plank Pose)
Intense stretch	Hip joint (flexion) (abduction) (ipsilateral)	-
Forward bend	Hip joint (extension) (contralateral)	-
-	Knee joint (flexion) (ipsilateral)	-
-	Knee joint (extension) (contralateral)	-
-	Spine (flexion)	-

Technique:

a. Start by assuming Bharmanasana (Table Top Pose).
b. Bend your elbows and place them directly under your shoulders. Ensure they are shoulder wide apart.
c. Inhale and slowly extend your legs back while aligning your head, shoulders, hips, and heels—similar to getting into a low plank position. Keep your neck, spine, and pelvis neutral.
d. Exhale and gently move your right leg (ipsilateral) forward, outside your right elbow, while the left leg (contralateral) remains extended.
e. Breathe normally and hold this position for about 3 to 10 breaths.
f. Repeat it for 3 to 5 times on each side.

Benefits

- Helps release tight hip muscles
- Mobilises the hip joint and increases its range of motion
- Improves flexibility of the spine and hips
- Helps prevent dead butt syndrome
- Can contribute to balance and stability
- Strengthens the shoulder, arms, and chest muscles
- Cuts body fat, especially when practised in a movement-oriented yoga class
- Promotes pelvic floor muscle health
- Relieves mild back pain
- Releases the inner thigh and groin muscles

Common Mistakes to Avoid

- Moving your extended leg
- Rounding your back
- Bending the knees above or below 90 degrees
- Skipping warm-up
- Lifting the hip beyond your shoulders

Biomechanics

Keep your neck (cervical spine) aligned with the rest of the spine. There's no need to look forward.

In Lizard Pose, the glutes on the opposite side of the body contract to extend the hip, while the gluteus maximus on the same side as the bent knee stretches. Keep the bent knee close to your body to further relax and stretch the gluteal muscles.

The hip joint, being the second most mobile joint, is a ball and socket joint with about 360 degrees of range of motion. It sacrifices stability for mobility.

Utthan Pristhasana helps stretch the muscles and connective tissues in and around the hip region, contributing to both stability and mobility.

If possible, let your front leg bear about half of the total load. The rest of the weight can be supported by the forearms and the rear leg. In this position, the front quadriceps muscle stabilises, while the back quadriceps muscle extends the knee.

Do not force hip squaring; let the pelvic movement be natural. Make sure to engage your core muscles to protect your spine. This will also allow your back muscles to release even more. Additionally, this engagement enables the quadratus lumborum, spinal erectors, and latissimus dorsi to stretch actively, contributing to a stable trunk area.

Lastly, allow the scapulas to protract; this will activate the underactive serratus anterior muscles.

Modifications

- **Regression I:** If you feel the stretches are too intense, regress by lowering the extended (opposite side) knee.
- **Regression II:** Another way to regress is by extending both elbows. This will decrease the intensity of the stretches and can also be combined with Regression I.
- **Progression:** If you want to deepen the stretch, try pushing the knee further away from the body, or place your hand on the same side as the knee and push it away from the body.
- **Prop Work:** You can use a yoga bolster or block under your extended knee to regress the stretch.

Anjaneyasana (Low Lunge Pose) and Ashwa Sanchalanasana (Equestrian Pose)

Etymology: *Anjaney* is Lord Hanuman's name; *Ashwa* means horse; *Sanchalan* is conduction; *Asana* means pose.

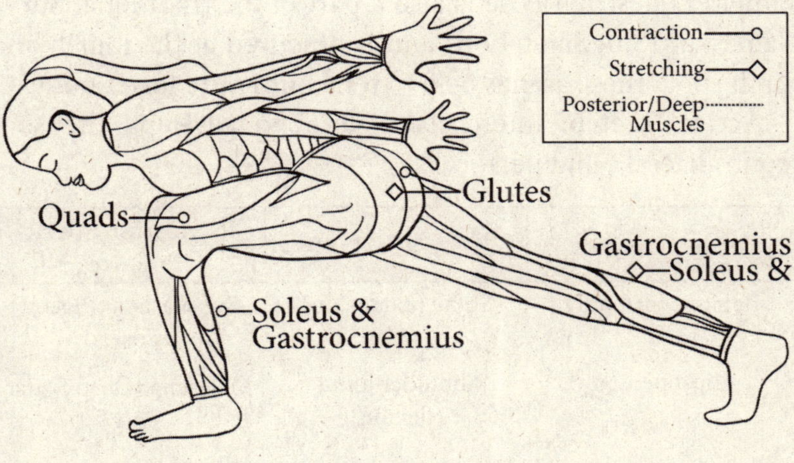

Anjaneyasana

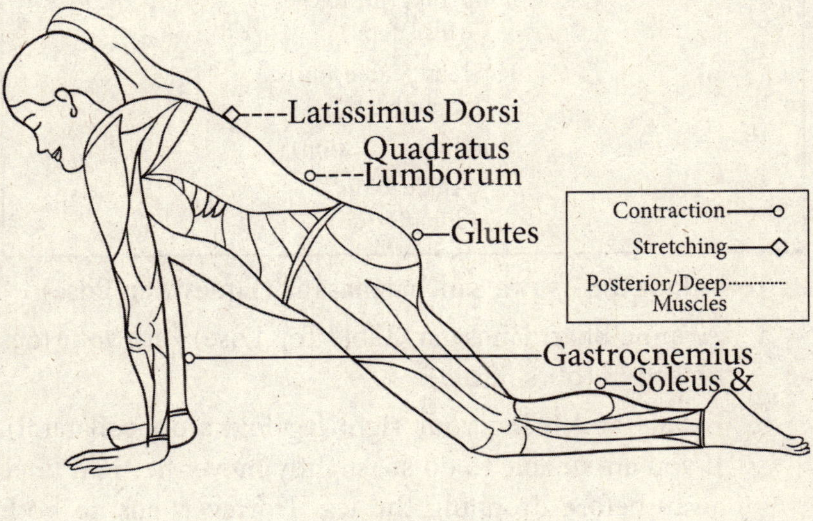

Sanchalanasana

The Anjaneyasana or Low Lunge Pose is named after Lord Hanuman as he was the son of Mother Anjani. Ashwa Sanchalanasana (Equestrian Pose) resembles Anjaneyasana. The only difference between Ashwa Sanchalanasana and Anjaneyasana is the placement of arms, everything else is similar. Equestrian Pose is also a part of the traditional Surya Namaskar (Sun Salutation) and is practised at the fourth and ninth spot. These asanas help to tone our entire lower body.

Active Stretch: Intercostals, glutes, quadriceps, iliopsoas (contralateral), and pectoralis.

Asana Category	Targeted Area	Preparatory Yogic Practices
Beginner-friendly	Spine (extension)	Kapotasana (Pigeon Pose)
Hip-opening	Shoulder joints (flexion)	Malasana (Deep Squat Pose)
Chest/heart opening	Elbow joints (extension)	-
-	Hip joint (flexion) (ipsilateral)	-
-	Hip joint (extension) (contralateral)	-
-	Knee joints (flexion)	-
-	Ankle joints (dorsiflexion)	-

Technique for Ashwa Sanchalanasana (Equestrian Pose):

a. Assume Bharmanasana (Table Top Pose) with your toes tucked in (dorsiflexed).

b. Exhale and bring your right leg forward (ipsilateral). If you are unable to do so, slightly move the right knee away before dropping the leg. However, ensure both ankles, knees, and hips are in their respective alignment.

c. Continue exhaling and slightly move your right knee forward and rear leg back. This will provide a gentle stretch in and around your hip muscles.
d. Inhale and either maintain your hands in place or extend your spine slightly backwards while raising your arms.
e. Technique for Anjaneyasana (Low Lunge Pose or Cresent Lunge Pose):
f. Exhale and from the Equestrian Pose, gently extend your rear leg. Meanwhile, maintain your front leg at about 90 degrees.
g. Inhale and extend your arms up or keep them as they are.
h. Breathe normally and hold this asana for about 5 to 10 breaths.
i. Repeat 3 to 5 times on each side.

Benefits

- Helps release tight pelvic muscles
- Stretches the abdominal, chest, and gluteal muscles
- Strengthens the hamstring, back, and shoulder muscles
- Can release negative emotions
- Prepares for more advanced asanas
- Can relieve discomfort during menstruation
- Improves the range of motion of the joints

Common Mistakes to Avoid

- Bending the front knee beyond comfort
- Keeping the ankles in an incorrect position
- Arching the neck beyond comfort

- Gazing upwards
- A steep backbend

Biomechanics

The gluteal muscles engage to extend the contralateral leg back, while the antagonist to the glutes, the contralateral iliopsoas stretches. Meanwhile, the hamstrings contract, allowing the knees to lower.

In the ipsilateral leg, the iliopsoas muscles flex the hip joint, while the glutes stretch. At the same time, the quadriceps muscle acts against as it lengthens, and the hamstring muscle stabilises the movement by contracting.

In both legs, the tibialis anterior muscles contract along with the peroneal muscles (longus and brevis) to maintain balance and flex the ankle joints. This stretches the soleus muscles and gastrocnemius muscles.

The trapezius muscles contract along with the spine erectors and the quadratus lumborum facilitates the backbend and stabilises the pelvis. This stretches the chest and abdominal muscles.

Anjaneyasana involves a more lifted stance than Ashwa Sanchalanasana. Therefore, the major difference between them is the extent of closed kinetic chain (CKC) movement. Anjaneyasana has a lesser degree of CKC motion as compared to Ashwa Sanchalanasana, where the knees are more supported.

As we know, the triceps muscles extend the elbows, and the deltoid muscles help flex the shoulder joints. When we lift the arms up, the latissimus dorsi muscle also lengthens.

Modifications

- **Regression:** To regress, you can drop the knee of your rear leg and stretch the toes out (plantarflexion).
- **Progression:** To progress, you can extend the knee of your rear leg. You can also move the heel slightly back; doing so will help you stretch muscles further.
- **Prop Work:** Practitioners often complain about having short legs or being unable to bring the leg completely forward. For most people, I'm afraid it is due to belly fat rather than short arms. In such cases, or otherwise, you can use yoga blocks to place your hands. This will give you additional lift, allowing you to move your leg easily.

Hanumanasana (Hanuman's Pose/Splits Pose)

Etymology: Hanuman is Lord Hanuman; *Asana* means posture.

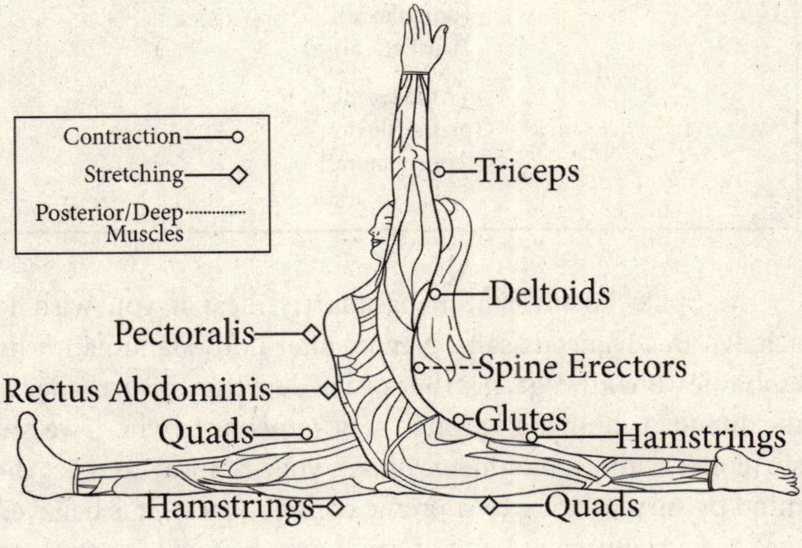

Hanumanasana

Asana Category	Targeted Area	Preparatory Yogic Practices
Sitting	Spine (extension)	Anjaneyasana (Low Lunge Pose)
Advanced	Shoulder ioints (flexion)	Ashwa Sanchalanasana (Equestrian Pose)
Hip opening	Elbow joints (extension)	Utthan Pristhasana (Lizard Pose)
-	Hip joint (flexion) (ipsilateral)	-
-	Hip joint (extension) (contralateral)	-
-	Knee joints (extension)	-
-	Ankle joint (dorsiflexion) (ipsilateral)	-
-	Ankle joint (plantarflexion) (contralateral)	-

The Splits Pose (Hanumanasana) is ideal if you wish to achieve an advanced asana. Named after Lord Hanuman, who embodies Bhakti yoga, it is the yoga of devotion or surrender to the divine. As humans, we often seek someone to whom we can surrender without judgment. Bhakti yoga is a way to relax the mind by surrendering to supreme consciousness. It is believed that Lord Hanuman is one of the divine beings who attained *Ashta Siddhis* (eight accomplishments) as suggested by the legendary yogic scripture Patanjali Yoga Sutra. Hanumanasana, an advanced asana, requires significant hip joint mobility and supple muscles.

Active Stretch: Intercostals, glutes (ipsilateral), rectus abdominis, iliopsoas (contralateral), pectoralis, gastrocnemius, and soleus (ipsilateral).

Technique:

a. Assume Bharmanasana (All Fours or Table Top Pose) with your toes tucked in (dorsiflexed).
b. Exhale and bring your right leg forward (ipsilateral). If you cannot do so, slightly move the right knee outward before lowering it. However, ensure that both ankles, knees, and hips are properly aligned.
c. Continue exhaling and move your right knee slightly forward and your rear leg slightly back. This will give you a gentle stretch in and around the hip muscles.
d. Breathe normally and gradually move your ipsilateral leg forward while extending the contralateral leg's knee straight. Hold this position for 5 to 10 breaths, remaining mindful of the stretches.
e. Now, reverse the movement. Bend your rear leg while fully extending the front leg. Hold this position for 5 to 10 breaths, remaining mindful of the stretches.
f. (Practise the previous two positions for 2 to 6 weeks, progressing gradually without seeking instant results.)
g. Continue breathing normally and once you reach the final pose, you can lift your arms towards the ceiling while keeping your spine erect.

h. Hold this asana for 3 to 10 breaths, repeating it 3 times on each side.

Benefits

- Improves the hip mobility
- Stretches the intercostal muscles
- Helps release tight muscles in the legs
- Can prevent spinal injuries
- Stretches the muscles of the legs, hips, and trunk
- Stretches the pelvic floor muscles
- Can improve reproductive health
- Can help redirect reproductive energies
- Can ease the mind.

Common Mistakes to Avoid

- Continuing this asana despite feeling pain
- Extending the knees beyond comfort
- Positioning the ankles incorrectly
- Arching the neck and gazing upwards

Biomechanics

Avoid forcefully stretching your legs, as this may cause excessive strain on your hips. One side of the body is usually tighter than the other, which is completely normal. Try to keep your hips squared, but don't force it; allow it to happen naturally.

In Hanumanasana, both legs work in almost opposing ways. The ipsilateral hip joint is flexed by the iliopsoas muscles, while the quadriceps and anterior tibialis muscles contract. This stretches the glutes, hamstrings, gastrocnemius, and soleus muscles in the ipsilateral leg. Conversely, in the contralateral leg, the gluteal muscles engage to extend it back, and the iliopsoas stretches. Meanwhile, the hamstring muscles contract slightly.

The erector spinae, transversospinalis, quadratus lumborum, and trapezius muscles contract to keep the spine erect, stretching the chest and abdominal muscles. Meanwhile, the external and internal oblique muscles stretch as they stabilise the torso. The deltoids flex the shoulders, while the triceps brachii muscles keep the elbows extended.

Modifications

- **Regression:** To regress, you can bend your front knee (ipsilateral).
- **Progression:** To progress, you can place your palms in front, stretching your hamstring muscles further.
- **Prop Work:** You can also use yoga blocks under both hands. This helps you manually adjust the stretch with your arms.
- **Prop Work:** You can place a rolled yoga blanket or bolster under your front thigh. This will limit your range of motion while allowing you to experience gentle stretches.

16

Strengthening Asanas: A Key Component for Holistic Health

Strengthening asanas are essential for every yoga practitioner. These asanas work on various muscles simultaneously, contributing to better joint stability, injury prevention, improved bone mineral density, and more. For an effective yoga practice, every sequence should include strengthening asanas. They can help heal emotional turmoil and make us more self-assured.

Virabhadrasana-I (Warrior-I Pose)

Etymology: *Vira* translates to warrior; *Bhadra* means friend; *Asana* means pose.

For perfect lower body conditioning, Virabhadrasana I is an ideal pose. It is often integrated into strength-based Vinyasa and Hatha yoga sessions, making it a staple in many sequences. It is definitely among the postures that attract angry looks from practitioners asking for a rest, much to the chagrin of yoga teachers. I have been there and have experienced it myself; however, when we relax in Shavasana, we realise it was all worth it.

Furthermore, despite its intensity, it is comparatively easier to perform, falling under beginner-friendly asanas.

Active Stretch: Glutes (ipsilateral), rectus abdominis, iliopsoas, and adductors.

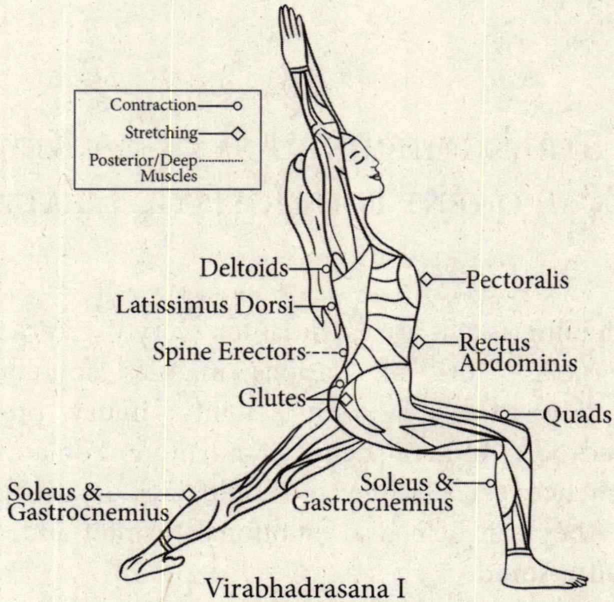

Virabhadrasana I

Asana Category	Targeted Area	Preparatory Yogic Practices
Beginner-friendly	Spine (extension)	Anjaneyasana (Low Lunge Pose)
Strengthening	Shoulder joints (flexion)	Virabhadrasana-II (Warrior-II)
Standing	Elbow joints (extension)	-
Balancing	Hip joints (abduction)	-
-	Knee joint (flexion) (ipsilateral)	-
-	Knee joint (extension) (contralateral)	-
-	Ankle joint (neutral) (ipsilateral)	-
-	Ankle joint (dorsiflexion) (inversion) (contralateral)	-

Technique:

a. Begin from Samasthiti (Equal Standing Pose).

b. Step your right leg forward (ipsilateral), about 3–4 feet apart from the left leg (contralateral). Ensure both feet are firmly placed on the yoga mat. For this, you may need to invert and externally rotate your left leg (usually at 45 degrees). According to some traditions, both of your heels should be in one line

c. Exhale and bend your right leg at a right angle and bring your right thigh almost parallel to the ground. The left leg will remain extended. If you can, square off your hips towards the front.

d. Inhale and flex your shoulders in front and bring your arms overhead, parallel to each other, or assume Namaskar Mudra (salutation gesture).

e. Breathe normally and hold this pose for about 3 to 10 breaths or according to your capacity.

f. Repeat 3 to 5 times on each side.

Benefits

- Helps strengthen the leg muscles
- Can help improve balance
- Aids in maintaining an upright posture
- Can reduce the risk of falls in seniors
- Promotes a better range of motion in the joints
- Isolates key leg muscles, which can help train both legs correctly
- Stretches the hip flexors or iliopsoas muscles

- Can improve focus
- Releases tight chest muscles

Common Mistakes to Avoid

- Wobbling
- Any noticeable tilt of the pelvis to any side
- Arching your back
- Gazing upwards or tilting your head
- Crossing your front knee over your front ankle

Biomechanics

Ensure you maintain a larger base of support for better stability. In this pose, the front quadriceps muscle (ipsilateral) contracts while lengthening against gravity to sustain the motion. Similarly, the rear leg is also extended by the quadriceps muscle. However, the front leg is likely to experience fatigue because it is lengthening while contracting.

When we extend our knee, it performs slight medial rotation. However, in asanas like Warrior I, the rear leg is already in external rotation. Therefore, these two opposing forces can create a torsion force on the knee. To prevent this, I suggest keeping a micro-flex in the rear knee.

The adductor muscles adduct the rear left leg, while the tensor fascia lata and gluteal muscles abduct the front leg.

The peroneal muscles help stabilise the soles of both feet and contribute to the stability of the ankle joints, preventing sprains.

The erector spinae and quadratus lumborum muscles work together to stabilise the pelvis and prevent excessive tilt. Meanwhile, the erector spinae and transverse abdominis muscles also help keep the spine upright while safeguarding it.

Lastly, the serratus anterior muscles help stabilise the scapulae when we lift the arms. The deltoid muscles assist in lifting the arms.

Modifications

- **Regression:** If you lose balance easily, instead of forming a line between your heels, place them on one of the diagonals of a wide rectangle. Doing so increases the base of support.
- **Progression:** If you wish to progress into the balance aspect of the asana, you can choose to internally rotate your rear leg and balance only on the toes of the rear and front feet. Doing so decreases the base of support, making it more challenging.
- **Wall Support:** Warrior I can also be practised with wall support, preventing imbalance.

Virabhadrasana II (Warrior II Pose)

Etymology: *Vira* means warrior; *Bhadra* translates to friend; *Asana* means posture.

How can Virabhadrasana II help improve cardiovascular system response? This pose primarily targets the legs. The arm and leg muscles are among the largest muscles of the body. When upper and lower limbs are moved for a longer range, it results in improved cardiovascular system response and heat generation. This heat signifies that the stored energy is being used, which burns extra calories.

Active Stretch: Gluteus maximus (ipsilateral), peroneus, and adductors.

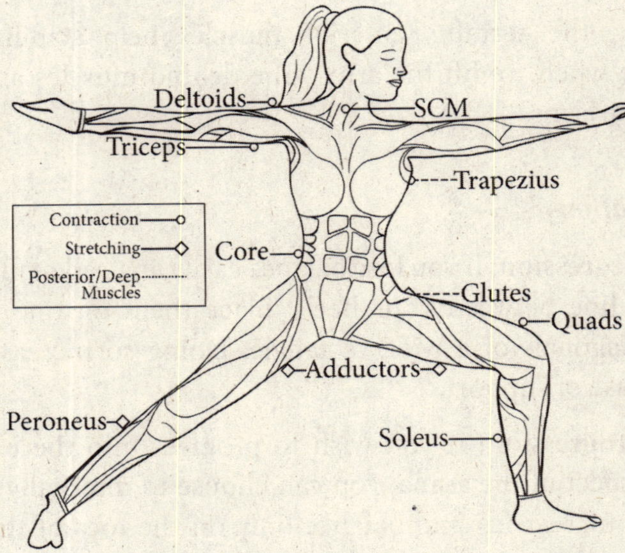

Virabhadrasana II

Asana Category	Targeted Area	Preparatory Yogic Practices
Beginner-friendly	Spine (extension)	Anjaneyasana (Low Lunge Pose)
Strengthening	Shoulder joints (abduction)	Utthita Tadasana (Five-Pointed Star Pose)
Standing	Hip joints (abduction)	-
-	Knee joint (flexion) (ipsilateral)	-
-	Knee joint (extension) (contralateral)	-
-	Ankle joint (neutral) (ipsilateral)	-
-	Ankle joint (dorsiflexion) (inversion) (contralateral	-

Technique:

a. Assume Samasthiti (Equal Standing Pose).
b. Bring your legs about 3 to 4 feet apart. Turn your right toes towards your right side (ipsilateral), meanwhile, turn your left one slightly inwards (about 45 degrees).
c. Inhale and abduct your arms till they reach shoulder level. Spread your fingers out.
d. Exhale and bend your right knee at about a 90-degree angle or to your comfort level.
e. Breathe normally and turn your head to the right.
f. Continue to breathe normally and hold this position for about 3 to 10 breaths or as long as you feel comfortable.
g. After completing one round, follow the instructions in reverse to revert to the starting position.
h. Repeat the same 3 to 5 times on each side.

Benefits

- Helps improve blood circulation
- Can aid in losing excess weight
- Strengthens leg muscles against gravity
- Tones muscles
- Can promote sound sleep
- May enhance the perception of happiness
- Can help prevent knee injuries
- Improves mindfulness
- Helps establish a connection with the self
- Stretches the adductor muscles
- Can boost stamina

Common Mistakes to Avoid

- Wobbling
- Any noticeable tilt of the pelvis to one side
- Mismatched arm movements
- Neglecting hip joint mobility

Biomechanics

In this pose, the front quadriceps muscle (ipsilateral) works against gravity to sustain the motion, while the quadriceps muscle in the contralateral leg assists with leg extension. However, fatigue is more likely to occur in the front leg, as it lengthens while contracting.

The erector spinae and quadratus lumborum muscles stabilise the pelvis and prevent excessive tilt. Simultaneously, the erector spinae and transverse abdominis muscles contract to maintain an upright spine and provide support.

The peroneal muscles help stabilise the soles of both feet, contributing to ankle joint stability and preventing sprains. The deltoid muscles play a crucial role in shoulder abduction, while the triceps brachii muscles extend the elbow joints, providing a gentle stretch to the biceps brachii.

In Warrior II Pose, it is challenging to maintain square hips. The turning of the head results from coordination between the sternocleidomastoid (contralateral) and splenius (ipsilateral) muscles.

Modifications

- **Regression:** If you experience discomfort in your inner thighs, you may reduce the distance between your legs.
- **Progression:** To deepen this asana, you can increase the distance between your legs. Doing so will place greater stress on the quadriceps muscles, but avoid overstraining.

- **Prop Work:** You may use a yoga chair under your bent knee to support the thigh.

Utkata Konasana or Deviasana (Goddess Pose)

Etymology: *Devi* means goddess; *Utkata* translates to ardent or fierce; *Kona* means angle; *Asana* means pose,

Utkata Konasana is interesting as it activates our powerful gluteal and leg muscles. We have three gluteal muscles—gluteus maximus, medius, and minimus. The gluteus maximus is the largest and contributes to significant power generation. Likewise, the remaining two gluteal and quadriceps muscles produce exceptional power to sustain such a complex motion. It is also known as the Deviasana, and the name 'Goddess Pose' originates from it. This intermediate asana can also be practised dynamically, making it a super-functional *sukshma vyayama*.

Active Stretch: Iliopsoas, adductors, and hamstrings.

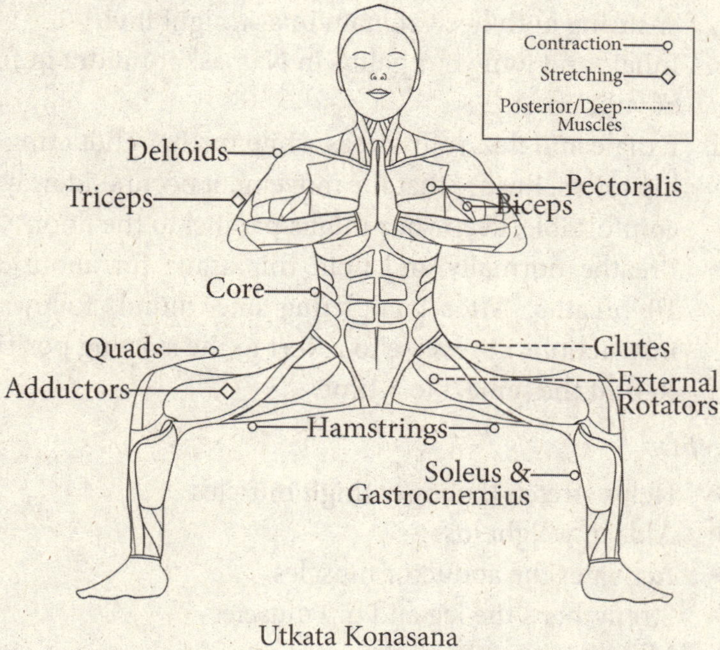

Utkata Konasana

Asana Category	Targeted Area	Preparatory Yogic Practices
Intermediate	Spine (extension)	Utkatasana (Chair Pose)
Standing	Shoulder joints (flexion) (internal rotation)	Malasana (Squat Pose)
Hip-opening	Elbow joints (flexion)	Utthan Pristhasana (Lizard Pose)
Inner thigh stretch	Hip joints (abduction)	-
-	Knee joints (flexion)	-
-	Ankle joints (neutral)	-

Technique:

a. Assume Samasthiti (Equal Standing Pose).
b. Exhale and bring your legs about 3 to 4 feet apart. Externally rotate your hip joints to about 90 degrees, ensuring both heels remain in a straight line.
c. Inhale and join your palms in Namaskar mudra in front of your chest.
d. Exhale and flex your knees while further abducting the hip joints. Ensure that the movement occurs sideways. If comfortable, keep your thighs parallel to the floor.
e. Breathe normally and hold this asana for about 3 to 10 breaths. After completing one round, follow the instructions in reverse to revert to the starting position.
f. Repeat the same 3 to 5 times.

Benefits

- Helps stretch the inner thigh muscles
- Aids in weight loss
- Activates the abductor muscles
- Strengthens the leg and hip muscles
- Mobilises the hip joints

- Can prevent dead butt syndrome
- Benefits individuals with a sedentary lifestyle
- Enhances blood circulation
- Can improve pelvic muscle functioning
- Can boost the reproductive system
- Can assist during pregnancy (second trimester)
- Believed to support menstrual health
- Protects the spine from injuries

Common Mistakes to Avoid

- Having too little or too much gap between the legs
- Tilting your body to either side
- Irregular or asymmetrical flexion of the knees
- Deep flexion of the knees
- Moving forward or backward
- Rounding or arching your back
- Not mobilising your joints before practice

Biomechanics

Almost all movements in this asana should occur in the frontal plane, with minimal forward and backward movements in the sagittal plane. Shifting forward or backward may indicate tight gluteal muscles.

Hip abduction is primarily facilitated by the gluteus medius and gluteus minimus muscles, while initial external hip rotation is performed by the piriformis, gemellus, and obturator internus muscles. However, after reaching the peak pose, these external rotator muscles experience a stretch.

To counter gravity, the quadriceps muscles, with the hamstrings, actively sustain knee flexion. Additionally, ensure that you maintain a square pelvis.

The adductor muscles—in the inner thigh area—act as antagonists to the hip abductor muscles (agonists). According to the principle of reciprocal innervation, our adductor muscles are stretched when we assume the Goddess Pose.

In each posterior leg compartment, large muscles such as the soleus, gastrocnemius, and peroneus (longus and brevis) help stabilise the body and legs.

To keep the spine upright and pelvis stable, various muscles work together—including the erector spinae, transversospinalis, transverse abdominis, rectus abdominis, quadratus lumborum, trapezius, and weakly the latissimus dorsi muscles.

To assume Anjali Mudra, we primarily activate the deltoid, biceps brachii, and pectoralis muscles.

Modifications

- **Regression:** If stretches are too intense, try narrowing the gap between your legs.
- **Progression:** To deepen the stretches, try widening your leg stance.
- **Prop Work:** Using a yoga belt or resistance band around your legs can help activate the gluteal muscles further.
- **Modification:** Abduct your shoulders and flex your elbows symmetrically with your legs. This will help activate your latissimus dorsi more effectively.

Phalakasana or Kumbhakasana (Plank Pose)

Etymology: *Phalak* translates to a wooden board; *Kumbhak* means holding (or holding the breath); Asana means pose.

Plank Pose needs no introduction. It is particularly popular among those who engage in resistance training. The power required to sustain this asana is remarkable, as a multitude of muscles engage in a series of co-contractions. Moreover, it can enhance stamina, supporting us in going the extra mile in life.

Active Stretch: Deltoids and rhomboids.

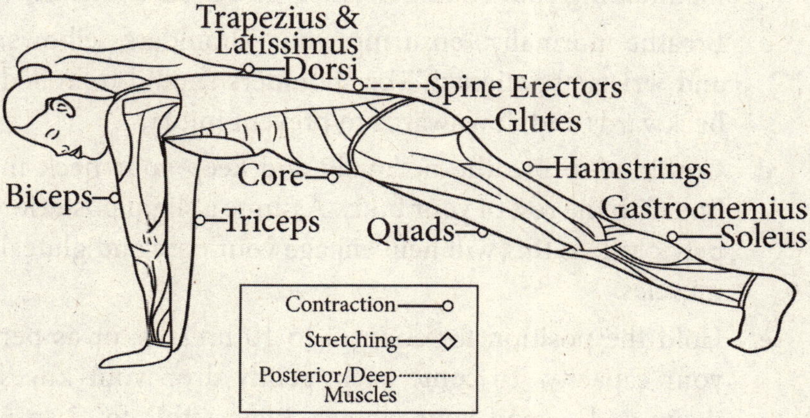

Phalakasana

Asana Category	Targeted Area	Preparatory Yogic Practices
Intermediate	Spine (slight flexion)	Bharmanasana (Table Top Pose or All Fours)
Intense	Shoulder joints (flexion)	Makara Adho Mukha Svanasana (Dolphin Plank Pose)
Strengthening	Elbow joints (extension)	Downward Facing Dog (Adho Mukha Svanasana)
-	Pelvis (slight posterior pelvic tilt)	-
-	Hip joints (extension)	-
-	Knee joints (extension)	-
-	Ankle joints (dorsiflexion)	-

Technique:

a. Begin by assuming Bharmanasana (Table Top Pose).

b. Inhale and slowly extend your legs back while maintaining your shoulders, hips, and heels in one line.

c. Breathe normally, ensuring your shoulders, elbows, and wrists are aligned. The shoulders should be rolled backwards and downwards to prevent injury.

d. Continue to breathe normally and keep your neck in line with the rest of your body. Assume a slight posterior pelvic tilt, as this will help engage your core and gluteal muscles.

e. Hold the position for about 3 to 10 breaths, or as per your capacity. To come back, gently drop your knees down and extend your elbows. Repeat this for 3 to 5 times.

Benefits

- Enhances overall appearance
- Can aid in burning calories
- An excellent form of body-weight resistance training
- Strengthens muscles in the arms, legs, torso, and back
- May increase resting metabolic rate (RMR)
- Prepares the body for inversions and strength-based yogic practices
- Can improve overall bone density
- Helps strengthen and protect joints
- May improve sleep quality

Common Mistakes to Avoid

- Elevating the shoulders
- Letting shoulders drop downwards
- Allowing hips to drop or lift
- Arching the back
- Extending the wrists beyond 90 degrees

Biomechanics

In Plank Pose, the serratus anterior muscles help to stabilise the scapula and prevent winging. For optimal activation, press your palms firmly downward, protract the scapula, and lift your upper body as high as possible.

Phalakasana is a closed kinetic chain exercise involving multiple muscles' co-contraction. Gripping the fingers with slight flexion protects the wrist joint by forming an arch in the palms, which activates additional forearm muscles. Additionally, pressing down with the entire palm, especially the heels, activates the triceps brachii and serratus anterior muscles.

A slight posterior pelvic tilt is advisable, as it helps engage the core and gluteal muscles effectively. The quadratus lumborum, transversospinalis, and erector spinae muscles work together to lift the back against gravity. The abdominal muscles counteract the transversospinalis and erector spinae muscles to maintain this pose.

The quadriceps help extend the knee, while the biceps femoris, part of the hamstring group, and the quadratus lumborum support the pelvis. Lastly, dipping the spine can place excessive strain on it, increasing injury risk, while lifting the spine may lead to ineffective muscle contractions.

Modifications

- **Regression**: If you wish to simplify this asana, try lowering your knees to the ground. This makes the pose significantly easier.
- **Progression**: To progress, ensure the correct engagement of all muscles and protraction of scapulae from the serratus anterior muscles.
- **Prop Work**: Use yoga blocks to improve your grip and support alignment.

Chaturanga Dandasana (Four-Limbed Staff Pose)

Etymology: *Chatur* means four; *Anga* translates to limb; *Danda* means staff or stick; *Asana* means posture.

Chaturanga Dandasana is also translated as the Four-Limbed Staff Pose and is commonly referred to as the 'Low Plank Pose'. The Chaturanga Dandasana is one of the more intense strength-based asanas. In this pose, many of our muscles contract to sustain a complex motion. It is particularly popular among practitioners of Vinyasa or flow-based yoga and is a vital part of various contemporary Surya Namaskar sequences.

Active Stretch: Deltoid, triceps brachii, and rhomboids.

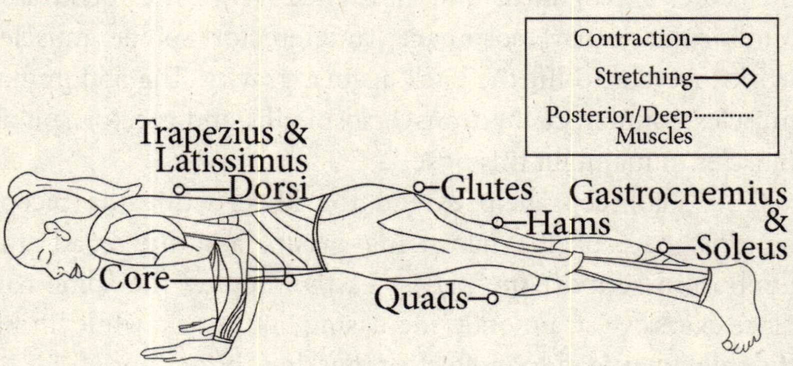

Chaturanga Dandasana

Asana Category	Targeted Area	Preparatory Yogic Practices
Intermediate	Spine (slight flexion)	Phalakasana (High Plank Pose)
Intense	Shoulder joints (extension)	Makara Adho Mukha Svanasana (Dolphin Plank Pose)
Strengthening	Elbow joints (flexion)	-
-	Pelvis (posterior pelvic tilt)	-
-	Hip joints (extension)	-
-	Knee joints (extension)	-
-	Ankle joints (dorsiflexion)	-

Technique:

a. Start by assuming Bharmanasana (Table Top Pose or All Fours).

b. Inhale and slowly extend your legs back while maintaining your shoulders, hips, and heels in one line. Additionally, your shoulders, elbows, and wrists should also align.

c. Exhale and bend your elbow joints to approximately a 90-degree angle by moving your shoulders forward without changing the position of your elbows. This way, your wrists and elbows will form a 90-degree angle with your shoulders. Ensure that your shoulders are rolled backwards and downward to prevent injuries.

d. Breathe normally and keep your neck aligned with the rest of your body. Assume a slight posterior pelvic tilt and engage your gluteal and abdominal muscles.

e. Continue to breathe normally and hold this position for about 3 to 10 breaths, or as per your capacity. To return, gently drop your knees down and extend your elbows. Repeat this 3 to 5 times.

Benefits

- Strengthens arms, back, abdomen, and leg muscles
- Helps to retain a healthy body
- Improves aesthetics
- Helps to prevent injuries
- Promotes a healthy spine
- Prepares for advanced yoga asanas
- Enhances everyday body posture
- Delays ageing by preserving elastin and collagen tissues

Common Mistakes to Avoid

- Dropping the shoulders forward
- Dropping or lifting the hips
- Arching the back
- Extending the wrists beyond 90 degrees
- Downward-facing shoulders

Biomechanics

In Chaturanga Dandasana, the serratus anterior muscles help to steady the scapulae and prevent winging. They are accompanied by the rhomboid muscles in stabilising the scapulae.

As this asana is intense on the shoulder joints, the rotator cuff muscles, biceps brachii, and deltoid muscles collectively help to stabilise the shoulder joint.

Chaturanga Dandasana is among the closed-kinetic chain (CKC) motions.

Activating the fingers can enhance the wrist protection mechanism. Thus, instead of keeping the palms flat, flex them. Effective palm engagement forms an arch in the palms and signals better activation of the triceps brachii and serratus anterior muscles.

The triceps brachii play a vital role in balancing the elbow. They work alongside the biceps brachii and brachialis muscles.

Many people suggest maintaining a neutral pelvis; however, in my opinion, a slight posterior pelvic tilt is better as it effectively engages the core and gluteal muscles, which can help prevent spinal injuries.

The quadratus lumborum, transversospinalis, and erector spinae muscles work in tandem to lift the back, while the abdominal muscles also work synergically with them to sustain the motion.

The pectoralis muscles also play a critical role in sustaining this pose. However, overactivation of the pectoralis muscles can contribute to downward-rotated shoulders, which should be avoided.

The biceps femoris of the hamstring group, along with the quadriceps and gluteal muscles, maintain the lift of the thighs and hips.

Modifications

- **Regression:** One way to regress into this pose is to drop your knee while maintaining the upper body in the same position.
- **Progression:** To progress, increase the number of breaths and the level of muscle contraction.
- **Prop Work:** Use yoga blocks under your palms to improve your grip.

17

Mastering Upside-Down Asanas

Upside-down asanas are also known as Viparita Karani Mudra (inversion asanas). These asanas are generally categorised by the position of the head below the heart level or the heart below the leg level. A common misconception surrounding these asanas is that they circulate more blood to the brain. However, in reality, this seldom occurs due to the blood-brain barrier, which prevents any undue number of substances from entering the brain. These asanas can contribute to improved body-mind coordination and spatial awareness, and help remove excess mucus from the lungs. In this chapter, read about each asana to learn more about their biomechanics in detail.

Adho Mukha Svanasana (Downward Facing Dog Pose)

Etymology: *Adho* means downward; *Mukha* means face; *Svan* translates to dog; *Asana* means pose.

Adho Mukha Svanasana resembles the stretch that dogs usually perform while facing downwards. In some yogic traditions, it is often referred to as Parvatasana (Mountain Pose), where *parvat* means mountain. This asana is also part of the traditional Surya Namaskar, occupying the eighth position in the sequence. Additionally, Adho Mukha Svanasana features in almost all other forms of Surya Namaskar. As an inversion, it positions the head below the heart level.

Active Stretch: Rectus abdominis, latissimus dorsi, glutes, and biceps brachii.

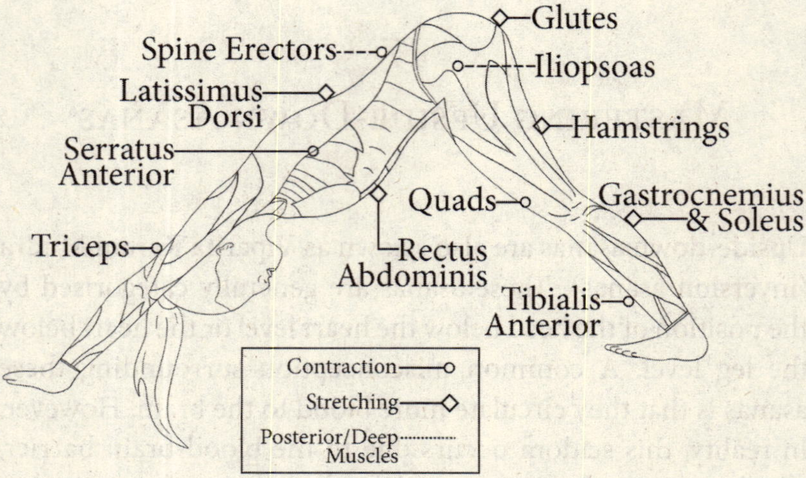

Adho Mukha Svanasana

Asana Category	Targeted Area	Preparatory Yogic Practices
Beginner-friendly	Spine (extension)	Balasana (Child Pose)
Forward bend	Shoulder joints (flexion)	Ardha Pincha Mayurasana (Dolphin Pose)
Inversion/upside-down	Elbow joints (extension)	Makara Adho Mukha Svanasana (Dolphin Plank Pose)
-	Hip joints (flexion)	Phalakasana (Plank Pose)
-	Knee joints (flexion)	-
-	Ankle joints (dorsiflexion)	-

Technique:

a. Assume Bharmanasana (Table Top Pose). Gently arch your back or assume an anterior pelvic tilt.

b. Exhale and spread your fingers outwards. Push your palms and toes onto the mat to generate a lift. Slowly lift your tailbone towards the ceiling. Your heels will also lift.

c. Breathe normally and keep your elbows slightly flexed. Relax your shoulders and keep them down.

d. Inhale and ensure your spine remains extended (lengthened). To prioritise this extension, you can bend your knees—by micro-flexing them.

e. Breathe normally and hold this position for about 3 to 10 breaths. In Vinyasa, we usually assume this for 5 breaths.

f. Repeat the instructions in reverse to return to the starting position and relax.

Benefits

- Helps fight inflammation (Arora et al, 2008)
- Contracts the chest, abdominal, and front thigh muscles
- Stretches hamstring, calves, and spine erector muscles
- Helps calm the mind
- Aids in overall mobility
- Boosts blood circulation
- Trains the spine and surrounding connective tissues
- Prepares for other inversion asanas and dynamic flows

Common Mistakes to Avoid

- Looking towards the navel

- Flexing or hunching the spine
- Dropping the heels, compromising the spine
- Hyperextending the elbows and knees
- Arching the back too much
- Pushing the shoulders beyond comfort
- Keeping too much or too little gap between arms and legs

Biomechanics

While it is common for yoga teachers to give cues, such as directing the gaze towards the navel, it is vital to understand that this can compromise cervical spine alignment.

The Adho Mukha Svanasana stretches the posterior chain of muscles, including the hamstrings, gastrocnemius, soleus, spinal erector muscles, and more. It also contracts the anterior chain of muscles, including the pectoralis, abdominals, quadriceps, tibialis anterior, iliopsoas, and others.

In this pose, it is advisable to maintain an anterior pelvic tilt, as this helps to keep the spine neutral, reduces load, and further stretches the back muscles. The latissimus dorsi muscles contribute to stability in this pose; however, they also internally rotate the shoulders, which can interact with the acromion process, potentially causing concern. To address this, begin by externally rotating the humerus bones until reaching the final pose, then gradually try internal rotation to stretch the shoulders.

The shoulder joint is among the less stable joints, so I recommend avoiding pressing it (inward or downward) beyond 180 degrees of flexion in this asana. It is also safer to shift the weight and motion towards the legs. To ensure shoulder safety, the scapulae should rest in their neutral position, attached to the ribcage (scapular depression). To achieve this, I suggest creating a strong lift by pressing through the entire arms—a good practice for yoga postures where the shoulders bear weight.

Lastly, in this asana, there may be slight internal rotation of the knees towards the medial side when extending them. This helps stabilise the lateral aspect of the knee joints.

Modifications

- **Regression:** If you are unable to maintain this pose correctly, feel free to bend your knees until your spine lengthens appropriately.
- **Regression II (Ardha Pincha Mayurasana or Dolphin Pose):** If the pose remains challenging, try this forearm version where, instead of using your palms, place your entire forearms on the mat. Everything else stays the same.
- **Progression:** If you wish to advance in this asana, you may rest your heels on the mat. However, if doing so compromises the neutrality of your spine, it is not advisable.
- **Prop Work:** For better grip, you may use two yoga blocks.

Bakasana (Crane Pose)

Etymology: *Baka* translates to crane; *Asana* means posture.

Bakasana is among one of the advanced yoga asanas. It is often confused with the Kakasana (Crow Pose), which is more suitable for intermediate yoga practitioners. Here, we will learn both these asanas while focusing mainly on the Bakasana.

Bakasana is an arm-balancing yoga asana, keeping the entire body weight on the arms. Thus, only the palms serve as the base of support. Several muscles intricately play their roles to sustain this motion.

Active Stretch: Quadriceps, latissimus dorsi, erector spinae, transversospinalis, glutes, and tibialis anterior.

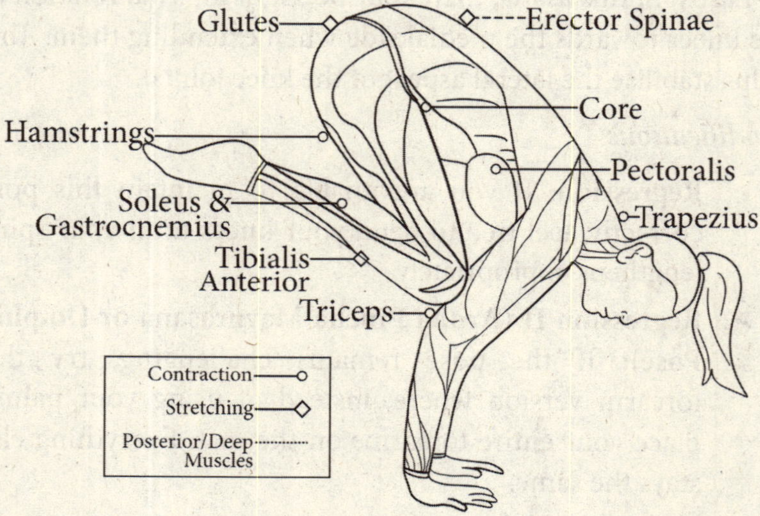

Bakasana

Asana Category	Targeted Area	Preparatory Yogic Practices
Advance	Spine (neutral)	Malasana (Squat Pose)
Inversion/ upside down	Shoulder joints (flexion) (internal rotation)	Kakasana (Crow Pose)
Arm balance	Elbow joints (extension)	Tulasana (Balance Pose)
Balancing	Pelvis (neutral)	-
Strengthening	Hip joints (extension) (adduction)	-
-	Knee joints (extension)	-

Technique for Kakasana (Crow Pose):

a. Start by getting into a deep squat position with your palms in front—on the floor, with a should-wide gap.
b. Spread and grip your fingers tightly on the mat. Gently bend your elbows slightly and move them outwards (internal rotation of the shoulders).
c. Shift your body weight on your palms.
d. Exhale and one by one load your knees on the outer edge of the elbows, specifically on your triceps.
e. Inhale and gradually shift your centre of gravity (or head) slightly forward. Keep your elbows extended. Engage your core as best as you can.
f. Breathe normally and hold this position for about 3 to 10 breaths.
g. Repeat the instructions in reverse to come back. Perform it 3 to 5 times.

Bakasana (Crane Pose):

a. In Crane Pose, unlike Kakasana, the knees rest on the socket of the underarms.
b. Exhale and extend your elbows fully and your knees partially by raising your heels from the squatting position. in a way that your knees can plug the underarms (underneath the glenohumeral joint).
c. Gradually, shift your centre of gravity (or head) slightly forward. Keep your elbows extended and engage your core as best as you can.
d. Inhale and one by one lift both feet.
e. Breathe normally and hold this position for about 3 to 10 breaths.

f. Repeat the instructions in reverse to return to the starting position. Perform this 3 to 5 times.

Benefits

- Helps engage and strengthen the core muscles
- Can help prevent backache
- Strengthens arm muscles
- Tones key muscles
- Sets the groundwork for advanced arm-balancing postures
- Improves overall awareness levels
- Can enhance attention span
- Can help activate the facial muscles
- Enhances spatial awareness

Common Mistakes to Avoid

- Not mobilising the joints
- Straining the wrist joint
- Practising without proper guidance
- Practising on an uneven surface
- Not balancing the centre of gravity

Biomechanics

The Bakasana requires significant core and back muscle activation. Here, the core and back muscles play a crucial role in stabilising the entire body. The back muscles—including the lower and middle trapezius, erector spinae, and transversospinalis muscles—counteract gravitational pull by contracting while lengthening.

The core muscles, along with the iliopsoas, create space for the leg muscles and help maintain balance. Meanwhile, the hamstrings flex the knees, while the soleus and gastrocnemius muscles plantarflex the ankles. In Bakasana, the triceps brachii, biceps brachii, and deltoid muscles are also essential for stabilising and supporting the load on the arms.

For better stability, keep the scapulae neutral (or slightly abducted) while resting on the ribcage by engaging the serratus anterior muscles. To activate the serratus anterior, push firmly into the floor with your arms.

Modifications

- **Regression (Kakasana):** For a simpler version of Bakasana, try Kakasana (Crow Pose). Here, instead of placing your knees under the glenoid fossa (the shoulder socket), rest the knees on the outer edge of the elbows with a slight bend in the elbows. The rest of the asana remains similar, but this small adjustment significantly eases core and back muscle engagement.
- **Progression (Eka Pada Bakasana):** For those looking to progress, try the one-legged variation, Eka Pada Bakasana. This pose is challenging as it maintains the same base of support as Bakasana, but with one leg extended. This adds difficulty and requires heightened muscle coordination.
- **Prop Work:** If balancing or lifting the body is challenging, try practising with a yoga block. The block increases height and enhances finger grip, which many individuals find helpful when assuming Bakasana.

Ardha Halasana (Half Plough Pose)

Etymology: *Ardha* means half; *Hal* translates to plough; *Asana* means pose or posture.

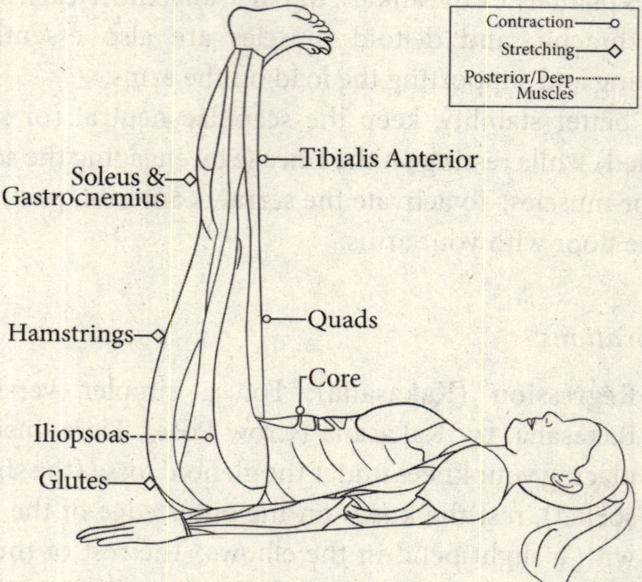

Ardha Halasana

Asana Category	Targeted Area	Preparatory Yogic Practices
Forward bend	Spine (flexion)	Dandasana (Staff Pose)
Beginner-friendly	Shoulder joints (extension)	Eka Pada Uttana Padasana (One-Legged Raised Leg Pose)
Core-centric	Hip joints (flexion)	Eka Pada Ardha Halasana (One-Legged Half Plough Pose)
Reclining/supine	Knee joints (extension)	Uttana Padasana (Raised Leg Pose)
Inversion/ upside down	Ankle joints (dorsiflexion)	-

Ardha Halasana is an asana that beginners can easily practise as long as there are no contraindications. It is primarily popular among yogis as a core-focused asana, requiring the coordinated effort of several abdominal muscles. The Ardha Halasana is often mistaken for Viparita Karani. While it may not seem like a full inversion, such as a Shoulder Stand or Headstand, it does involve a significant elevation of the legs. This makes it a beneficial practice for stimulating the body's systems and promoting calm, as it encourages blood flow to the heart and head.

Active Stretch: Glutes and hamstrings.

Technique:

a. Start by assuming Shavasana (Corpse Pose) or a simple supine position.
b. Join your legs and bring your arms by the sides, while the palms face the floor, and your ankle joints are pulled inwards.
c. Exhale and gently lift your legs, either simultaneously or one at a time, bringing them to a 90-degree position—perpendicular to the floor and upper body.
d. Breathe normally and hold this position for about 3 to 10 breaths.
e. Slowly and gradually rest your legs down on the mat. Repeat this 3 to 5 times.

Benefits

- Can improve overall posture in one's day-to-day life
- Promotes overall spinal health
- Can prevent spinal injuries
- Activates the core muscles

- Can prevent backache
- Activates the 'rest and digest' response
- Can improve gut health
- Helps relieve stress, anxiety, and depression
- Can improve mood disorders
- Provides mild stretches for the hamstring and calf muscles
- Prevents knee injuries
- Can be therapeutic for knee-related ailments

Common Mistakes to Avoid

- Hyperextending the knees
- Arching the lower back
- Lifting the waist or lower back
- Excessive pressure on the neck

Biomechanics

The Ardha Halasana follows the principle of the convex-concave rule. Here, the convex surface rolls over the concave surface. Therefore, compared to other forward bends, the motion here is simpler.

To sustain motion, it activates the iliopsoas and core muscles, including the transverse abdominis, rectus abdominis, external and internal oblique, and multifidus.

Ensure you maintain micro-flexion in your knee joints; doing so can prevent spinal arching and stretch the hamstring muscles more effectively.

In this asana, it is important to assume a posterior pelvic tilt. Our priority is the lumbar spine, which should be flattened on the ground instead of arched. An arched lower back can result in backache as the lumbar experiences compressive forces.

Ardha Halasana is an open kinetic chain movement. Therefore, if you practice it with yoga props, it will significantly decrease the contraction of the abdominal muscles.

Make sure to keep your core muscles activated throughout; however, this should not hinder the breathing cycle.

Modifications

- **Regression (Eka Pada Ardha Halasana):** One should test the waters before sailing; likewise, start with the one-legged variation of Ardha Halasana and then gradually proceed to the full Ardha Halasana.
- **Progression (Dynamic Eka Pada Ardha Halasana):** If you wish to progress into this asana, try the dynamic version of the Ardha Halasana. Here, practice Eka Padasana while altering the position of the legs, meaning that when one leg reaches the 90-degree angle, the other should be close to the floor. Keep alternating their positions.
- **Modification:** Ensure your lumbar spine is rested. If you cannot remove the arch, it is wise to place your palms underneath your hips; this will position the spine and pelvis into a posterior pelvic tilt, allowing the spine to flex.
- **Prop Work:** You can add a yoga blanket under your hips; doing so will help support your lower back.

Salamba Sirsasana (Supported Headstand)

Etymology: *Salamba* means supported or with support; *Sirsa* translates to head; *Asana* means pose or seat.

Sirsasana is also known as the Salamba Sirsasana. It is an inverted asana often considered advanced. People are often drawn to it for its impressive appearance. However, beyond

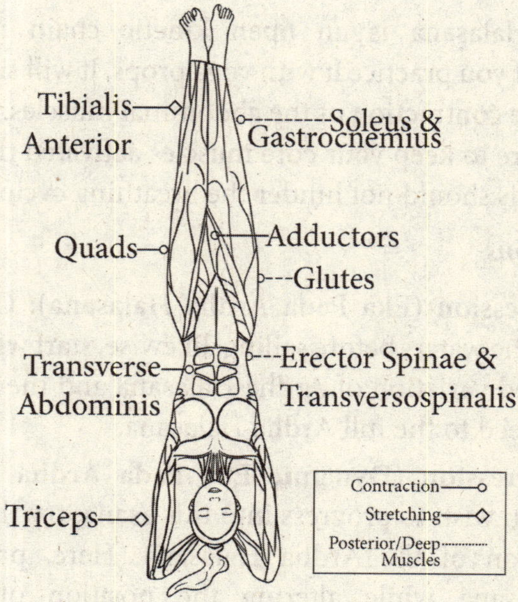

Salamba Sirsasana

Asana Category	Targeted Area	Preparatory Yogic Practices
Inversion/ upside-down	Spine (extension	Balasana (Child's Pose)
Advanced	Shoulder joints (flexion and abduction)	Makara Adho Mukha Svanasana (Dolphin Plank Pose)
Balancing	Elbow (flexion)	Chaturanga Dandasana (Four-Limbed Staff Pose)
-	Wrist joints (flexion)	Sarvangasana (Shoulder Stand Pose)
-	Pelvis (neutral)	-
-	Hip joints (extension)	-
-	Knee joints (extension)	-
-	Ankle joints (plantarflexion)	-

its aesthetics, Sirsasana offers several benefits, including the improvement of proprioception and equilibrioception. This pose challenges various parameters of the body including mental toughness, strength, resilience, coordination, and beyond.

Active Stretch: Triceps brachii and pectoralis.

Technique:

a. Assume Bharmanasana. Keep your breathing normal at almost all stages.
b. From here, press your elbows in the front, keeping a shoulder-wide gap.
c. Clasp your fingers in a way that your elbows and hands form an equilateral triangle. Assume that your elbows and clasped hands form three legs of a tripod. Grip them firmly on the mat.
d. Place the crown of your head on the yoga mat.
e. Gently extend your knees and bring your legs close to your upper body.
f. To balance the centre of gravity (like a see-saw), move your torso forward, and try to accommodate your folded legs.
g. Then, gently lift one leg while the other still touches the floor. Once you are well versed with the balancing factor (proprioception), lift the other leg as well.
h. Do not rush to extend your knees. Spend 2 to 3 seconds here.
i. Inhale and lift your legs one at a time.
j. Point your toes outwards.
k. Exhale and repeat the instructions in reverse to return to the starting position.
l. To relax, hold Balasana (Child's Pose) for a while.

Benefits

- Helps improve blood circulation throughout the body
- Enhances proprioception, which is the awareness of the body in an environment
- Increases overall strength
- Enhances neuromuscular coordination
- Believed to stimulate the functioning of the lymphatic system
- Can nourish the joints, ligaments, tendons, and cartilage

Common Mistakes to Avoid

- Arching the back
- Practising for too long
- Flexing the hips or pelvis beyond a comfortable range
- Practising without any guidance
- Making jerky movements
- Moving the neck
- Assuming asymmetrical positions

Biomechanics

Sirsasana does not increase blood circulation to the head. A barrier called the blood-brain barrier (BBB) protects the brain from external substances. The brain is a sophisticated part of our body that requires a constant blood supply and protection from the external environment, and the BBB ensures these conditions are met.

Ideally, your body should be upside down without much difference from the usual standing spinal stance. However, in this position, the cervical spine bears the entire body weight, which it is not designed to support. If we examine spinal anatomy, the cervical spine is the smallest of all, followed by the thoracic spine and lumbar spine. Therefore, holding Sirsasana for an extended period is not recommended.

For these reasons, arching or maintaining the spine in an asymmetrical position should be strictly avoided. Furthermore, to protect the spine and its delicate connective tissues, a yoga teacher should always assess this pose, prioritising a neutral spine.

Sirsasana requires intricate coordination among key muscles of the body, which work in sync to accomplish this asana. However, there's good news: Once you achieve it, your body will retain the 'muscle memory' of the pose. Therefore, after the initial attempts, it should become much easier. Still, safety must always be ensured.

Modifications

- **Regression:** A common way to learn Headstand Pose is to perform it with wall support. However, this should still be done under strict guidance. Begin by placing your legs on the wall, then release them one at a time. To protect your back, ask someone to stand on the opposite side to catch you if you fall.
- **Progression (Padma Sirsasana or Lotus Headstand):** Sirsasana can also be practised with lotus legs, known as Padma Sirsasana. However, this variation requires good mobility of the hip joints.
- **Prop Work:** I recommend using a thick mat while practising Sirsasana.

18

Finding Your Centre: The Science of Balance-Oriented Asanas

Balance-oriented asanas are more challenging than other asanas. While assuming these poses, we balance our body with a small base of support. Therefore, they engage our sense of balance and body awareness, known as equilibrioception and proprioception, respectively. Achieving these asanas provides a sense of confidence and satisfaction. Balance-oriented asanas epitomise the coordinated efforts of the brain, body, muscular system, and proprioceptors. We can divide them into arm-balancing asanas, leg-balancing asanas, and body-balancing asanas.

Vrksasana (Tree Pose)

Etymology: *Vrksa* translates to tree; *Asana* means pose or seat.

Vrksasana is a balance-oriented asana where the body is balanced on a single leg. According to ancient stories, several sages practised Vrksasana as part of their meditative practices. However, for most practitioners, practising its usual form is also very beneficial and sufficient. Additionally, it is believed that mastering this asana can lead to gaining enhanced focus.

Active Stretch: Obliques (ipsilateral), triceps brachii, rectus abdominis, and transverse abdominis.

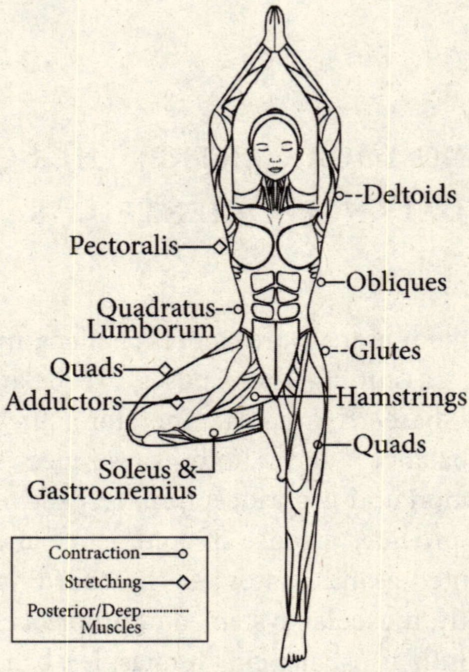

Vrksasana

Asana Category	Targeted Area	Preparatory Yogic Practices
Standing	Spine (neutral)	Samasthiti (Equal Standing Pose)
Balancing	Shoulder joints (flexion/abduction)	Tadasana (Palm Tree Pose)
Beginner-friendly	Elbow joints (flexion)	Urdhva Hastasana (Upward Salute)
-	Hip joint (extension) (contralateral)	-
-	Hip joint (abduction) (external rotation) (ipsilateral)	-
-	Knee joint (extension) (contralateral)	-
-	Knee joint (flexion) (ipsilateral)	-

Technique:

a. Begin by assuming Samasthiti (Equal Standing Pose).
b. Exhale and externally rotate and bend your right leg (ipsilateral). Hold your right ankle and place it on the superior part of your left thigh or close to your pelvis (contralateral). Continue exhaling and apply gentle pressure to your left thigh with your right foot and vice versa.
c. Inhale and gently join your palms in Namaskar Mudra in front of your chest or over your head.
d. Continue inhaling and grip the toes of your extended leg tightly on the mat.
e. Breathe normally and hold this asana for about 5 to 10 breaths.
f. Repeat the instructions in reverse to return to the starting position. Repeat this 3 to 5 times on each side.

Benefits

- Improves attention span
- Enhances overall awareness
- Improves spatial awareness
- Strengthens leg muscles
- Can improve the brain's cognitive abilities
- Improves overall balance and strength (Solakoglu, 2022).
- Can help improve overall bone density
- Can aid in preventing minor injuries
- Can help maintain the natural arch of the feet
- Trains the body in multiple planes of motion simultaneously

Common Mistakes to Avoid

- Excessive wobbling
- Losing focus
- Wearing slippery attire
- Not taking support upon losing balance
- Moving the bent knee

Biomechanics

This asana falls under the frontal plane. The quadratus lumborum muscles are vital in stabilising the pelvis. Without their support, the pelvic girdle may stoop lower than intended. A dropping pelvis could indicate that the quadratus lumborum cannot stabilise the pelvic girdle effectively.

Gripping the toes on the mat enhances leg muscle engagement, which, in turn, improves balance and stability; additionally, it helps protect the ankle joint from injury. Applying gentle pressure between the extended leg's thigh and the foot of the bent leg activates the adductor muscles and contributes to overall stability by forming a closed kinetic chain movement.

For those with shoulder injuries, it is advisable to practise this asana with Namaskar Mudra in front rather than raising the arm overhead. Raising the arms can place the shoulder articular capsules (essential for smooth motion) between the acromion process and the humerus. Namaskar Mudra also engages the pectoralis muscles in the chest.

To maintain balance, key leg muscles, including the peroneal, soleus, gastrocnemius, tibialis anterior, and tibialis posterior, work in unison. Additionally, the thigh and hip muscles of the extended leg, such as the gluteal, quadriceps, and adductor muscles, contribute significantly to stabilisation.

Maintaining a neutral spine involves cooperation between the erector spinae, transversospinalis muscles, and core muscles (abdominals).

Modifications

- **Wall Support:** If, despite proper instruction and practice, you are unable to perform the asana correctly, it may be due to your unique body structure, which is normal. In such cases, using wall support can be beneficial.
- **Variation I (Vrksasana with Open Arms):** Tree Pose is also often practised with open arms, as it is believed that this variation helps to attract positive energy.
- **Variation II (Vrksasana with Ardha Padmasana or Half Lotus):** In this variation, the folded leg is positioned in front of the extended leg's thigh.

Virabhadrasana III (Warrior III Pose)

Etymology: *Vira* means warrior; *Bhadra* translates to friend; *Asana* means pose or seat.

Virabhadrasana III is visually different from Virabhadrasana I (Warrior I Pose) and Virabhadrasana II (Warrior II Pose). In Warrior III, the focus shifts more towards balance. However, like the other two asanas, it also emphasises the lower limbs. As we know, the lower limbs support nearly all of our body weight and are among the body's primary weight-bearing structures. Therefore, working on these muscles is essential for promoting joint health.

Active Stretch: Hamstring (contralateral), gastrocnemius and soleus muscles (contralateral), glutes (contralateral), quadriceps muscle (ipsilateral), and iliopsoas muscle (ipsilateral).

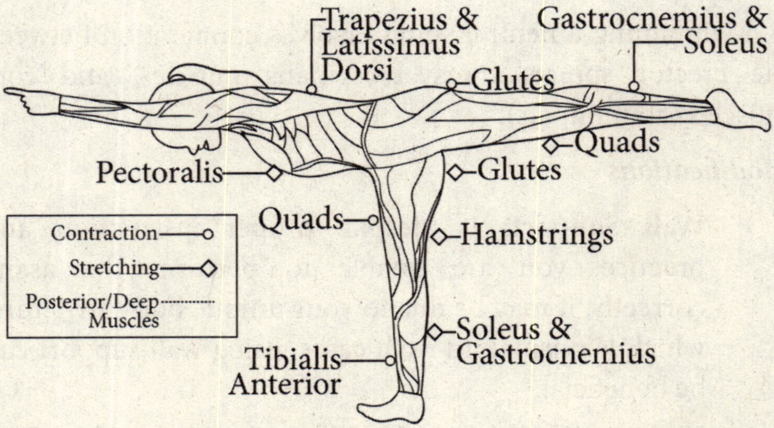

Virabhadrasana-III

Asana Category	Targeted Area	Preparatory Yogic Practices
Balancing	Spine (extension)	Virabhadrasana-I (Warrior-I Pose)
Strengthening	Shoulder joints (flexion)	Anjaneyasana (Low Lunge Pose)
Standing	Elbow joints (extension)	Vrksasana (Tree Pose)
Intermediate	Hip joints (extension) (ipsilateral)	-
-	Hip joints (flexion) (contralateral)	-
-	Knee joints (extension)	-
-	Ankle joints (dorsiflexion)	-

Technique:

a. Assume Samasthiti (Equal Standing Pose).

b Put your left leg (contralateral) forward—about 2 feet ahead of the right leg (ipsilateral). Now, flex your left knee slightly.

c. Slowly, lift your arms overhead.

d. With your left leg, grip your toes firmly on the mat and gradually shift your weight onto it.

e. Exhale and slowly move your entire body and right leg forward while keeping them aligned. Like a see-saw, lift your right leg and continue bending forward until your torso is parallel to the floor.

f. Inhale as your entire weight is placed on your left leg. Now, extend it with a micro-flex.

g. Breathe normally and hold this pose for about 3 to 10 breaths, or as per your capacity.

h. Repeat this 3 to 5 times on each side.

Benefits

- Activates the pelvic floor muscles
- Improves proprioception
- Enhances the mind-body connection
- Promotes mental stability
- Lifts mood
- Increases attention span
- Can encourage introspection
- Strengthens the lower limbs
- Strengthens the core and back muscles

Common Mistakes to Avoid

- Arching the back
- Locking the knees
- Leaning the torso towards the grounded leg
- Looking forward, as this may strain your neck
- Wobbling or making jerky movements

Biomechanics

The quadratus lumborum and erector spinae help stabilise the entire body, especially the pelvis and trunk. These muscles, along with the core, support spinal extension against gravity. The triceps brachii extend the elbow joints, while the deltoid muscles flex the shoulders. They also stabilise the shoulder joint and scapula alongside the serratus anterior, rotator cuff, trapezius, and rhomboid muscles.

To bear the body's weight on the grounded (contralateral) leg, the quadriceps and tibialis anterior muscles serve as prime movers, working with the hamstring, tibialis posterior, soleus, and peroneal muscles. In the lifted (ipsilateral) leg, the hamstring, soleus, and gastrocnemius muscles are the prime movers, working in conjunction with the quadriceps and tibialis anterior muscles.

The gluteal muscles extend the hip joint in the lifted leg while stabilising movement in the grounded leg. Hip flexion in the grounded leg is achieved by the iliopsoas (contralateral). The hip external rotators, iliopsoas, hip abductors, and external rotators (gluteus medius and minimus, and TFL) in the lifted leg maintain a neutral pelvis, keeping it parallel to the floor. Lastly, in the grounded leg, the gluteal and tensor fascia lata muscles prevent the pelvis from dropping.

Modifications

- **Regression:** Practise with arms by the sides of your body (shoulder extension) for greater control.
- **Prop Work:** For enhanced balance in Warrior III Pose, use two yoga blocks or a chair in front for support.
- **Wall Support:** Practise this asana with wall support if needed.

➢ **Progression:** To progress in this asana, lean the upper body slightly further forward.

Navasana (Boat Pose)

Etymology: *Nav* means boat; *Asana* translates to posture.

Named for its resemblance to a boat, Navasana is also known as Boat Pose. While often seen as a core-centric asana, it also strengthens the quadriceps, peroneal, and iliopsoas muscles. Navasana includes a balance component, activating the body's co-contraction mechanism, in which opposing muscles are engaged simultaneously. This pose is thought to improve the metabolic rate and may also prevent spinal conditions by strengthening the abdominal and back muscles.

Active Stretch: Glutes, hamstrings, tibialis anterior, quadratus lumborum, and rhomboids

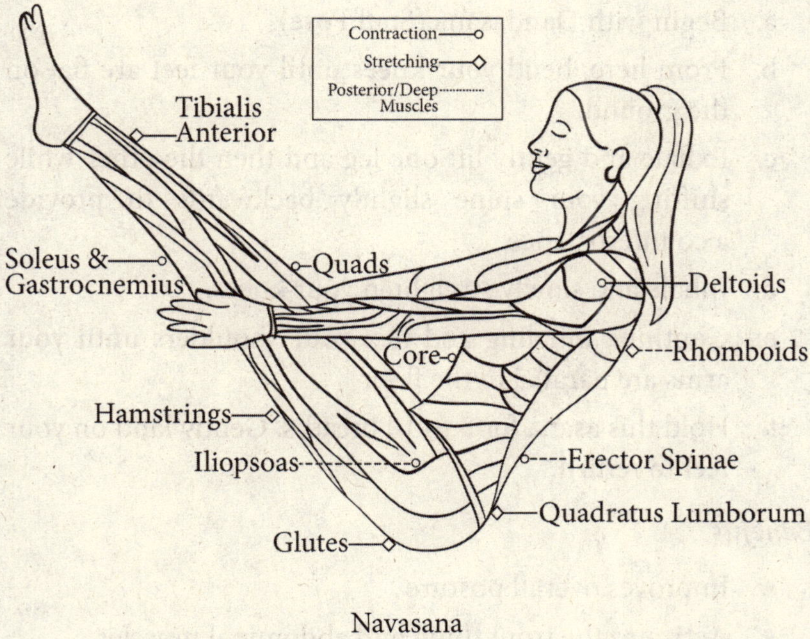

Navasana

Asana Category	Targeted Area	Preparatory Yogic Practices
Core-centric	Spine (slight flexion)	Dandasana (Staff Pose)
Balancing	Shoulder joint (flexion)	Ubhaya Padangusthasana (Both Big Toe Pose)
Forward bend	Lumbosacral joint (extension)	Ardha Uttanasana (Half Standing Forward Bend Pose)
Beginner-friendly	Hip joint (flexion)	-
-	Knee joint (extension)	-

Technique:

a. Begin with Dandasana (Staff Pose).
b. From here, bend your knees until your feet are flat on the ground.
c. Exhale and gently lift one leg and then the other while shifting your spine slightly backwards to provide a counterbalance.
d. Inhale and slowly straighten your knees.
e. Continue inhaling and flex your shoulders until your arms are parallel to the floor.
f. Hold this asana for 3 to 10 breaths. Gently land on your feet to return.

Benefits

- Improves overall posture
- Activates the front thigh and abdominal muscles

- Can improve neuro-muscular coordination
- Can aid in preventing back pain
- Increases intra-abdominal pressure, which aids digestion
- Can prevent spinal injuries.
- Strengthens the back muscles

Common Mistakes to Avoid

- Lifting the chest upwards
- Flexing the neck
- Arching the back

Biomechanics

This asana requires effective engagement of the abdominal muscles to prevent spinal discomfort. Boat Pose targets the quadriceps and abdominal muscles.

Avoid opening your chest intentionally, as this extends the spine and prevents effective engagement of the abdominal muscles. Keep your neck aligned with the rest of your spine—your chin slightly tucked in—or gaze towards your big toes.

The iliopsoas muscles are the primary movers responsible for hip flexion. They work in conjunction with the rectus abdominis, transverse abdominis, and quadriceps muscles to create the motion. The rectus and transverse abdominis muscles contract to slightly flex the trunk and support the spine against gravity, while the quadriceps muscles contract to lift the legs.

Due to shortened back muscles, you may occasionally experience slight discomfort in the back. To alleviate this, you can bend your knees.

The abdominal muscles, which act as trunk flexors, and the spinal erector muscles, which act as trunk extensors, contract together to ensure safe movement. Similarly, the gluteal muscles (hip extensors) and iliopsoas (hip flexors) also contract together. The quadriceps (hip flexor and knee extensor) and hamstrings (hip extensor and knee flexor) also work in tandem to create and sustain the motion. In short, these muscles co-activate in Navasana.

The deltoid muscles contract to flex the shoulder joints, while the triceps keep the elbows extended. The adductor muscles help draw the legs together, and the gastrocnemius and soleus muscles help to plantarflex the toes.

Modifications

- **Regression I:** If you experience difficulty assuming this asana, feel free to bend your knees.
- **Regression II:** You can also keep your hands grounded to avoid strain on your back, which greatly improves stability.
- **Progression:** To progress, you may lift your legs a little higher, which may require additional effort from your front thigh, hip flexor, and abdominal muscles.
- **Prop Work:** You can use a yoga strap in the middle of your feet, grasping it with your hands. This adjustment makes it a closed kinetic chain motion, making the pose easier to perform.

Adho Mukha Vrksasana (Handstand Pose)

Etymology: *Adho* translates to downward; *Mukha* means face, *Vrksa* is a tree; *Asana* means seat or pose.

Adho Mukha Vrksasana translates to Downward Facing Tree Pose; however, it is more popular as Handstand Pose or Full Arm Balance Pose. It is worth noting that apart from Adho Mukha Vrksasana, Vrschikasana (Scorpion Pose) is also often called Handstand Pose.

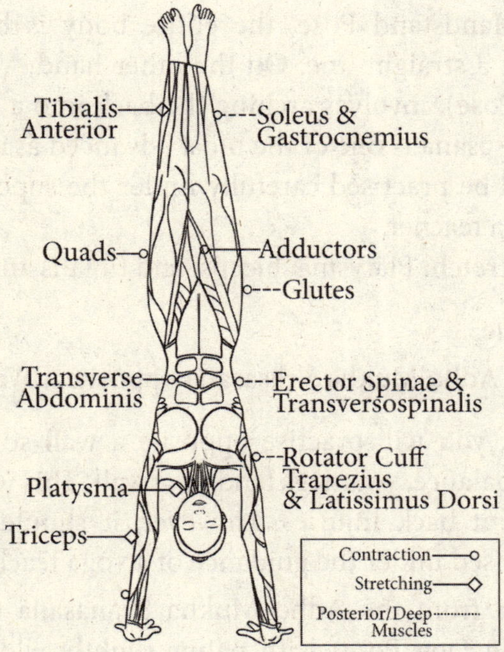

Adho Mukha Vrksasana

Asana Category	Targeted Area	Preparatory Yogic Practices
Advanced	Spine (neutral)	Sirsasana (Headstand Pose)
Inversion/ upside down	Shoulder joints (extension)	Pincha Mayurasana (Feathered Peacock Pose or Forearm Balance Pose)
Balancing	Elbow joints (extension)	Phalakasana (Plank Pose)
Strengthening	Pelvis (neutral)	-
-	Hip joints (extension)	-
-	Knee joints (extension)	-

In the Handstand Pose, the entire body is balanced on the arms in a straight line. On the other hand, Vrschikasana (Scorpion Pose), involves arching the back into a bend. Adho Mukha Vrksasana is one of the most advanced asanas in yoga, so it should be practised carefully under the supervision of a capable yoga teacher.

Active Stretch: Platysma, biceps, and tibialis anterior

Technique:

(Level 1: Adho Mukha Vrksasana opposite a Wall)

a. Here, you will practise opposite a wall so that if you lose balance, your legs land on a wall. This will also help prevent back injuries. However, it should be strictly practised under the guidance of a yoga teacher.
b. Begin from the Adho Mukha Svanasana (Downward Facing Dog Pose) with palms slightly wider than the shoulder level.
c. Slowly draw your legs close to your hands. Bring them even closer by lifting your heels. Meanwhile, bring your palms directly under your shoulders (shoulders flexion).
d. Tightly grip your fingers on the mat.
e. Fix your shoulder blades to their neutral position.
f. Take a few hops and try to engage your muscles to extend your legs towards the ceiling. The primary benefit of this level is that we have more control while landing back.
g. (Level 2: Adho Mukha Vrksasana without support)
h. Here, no wall support will be taken. This, too, must be practised under the guidance of a yoga teacher.
i. Inhale and gently activate your large back (trapezius, latissimus dorsi, and serratus anterior muscles) and

abdominal muscles, slightly hopping from one leg. See how far you can reach.

j. Breathe normally and stay at this level, gradually progressing further. Slowly, you will be able to lift both your legs up.

k. Hold this asana for about 3 to 10 breaths.

l. Gently come back by lowering your legs down with utmost muscular control.

Benefits

- Can improve neuromuscular coordination
- Enhances proprioception
- Strengthens the core, arm, spinal, and leg muscles
- Helps boost confidence
- Can aid in enhancing bone density
- Improves joint and connective tissue health
- Increases blood circulation
- Enhances lymphatic circulation
- Improves the immune system response
- Can shred excess fat
- Can enhance the resting metabolic rate

Common Mistakes to Avoid

- Going into a backbend
- Maintaining an inadequate gap between the arms
- Widening the arms beyond control
- Practising without proper guidance
- Not mobilising, resulting in injuries
- Moving the arms abruptly, resulting in injuries

- Hyperextending the elbow joints
- Making jerky movements

Biomechanics

Many individuals, especially those with hypermobility, are prone to adopting a backward extension stance, which should be avoided. Adho Mukha Vrksasana is designed to be a coordination-based strengthening asana, not a hypermobility-oriented one.

The elbows should be kept at approximately 180 degrees to ensure proper muscle engagement. The triceps brachii muscles play a vital role in this asana by stabilising the elbows while carefully working with the antagonists, namely the biceps brachii and brachialis muscles.

Like other inversion asanas, Adho Mukha Vrksasana is often thought to direct blood flow towards the head. However, this effect is limited by the blood-brain barrier (BBB), which protects the brain.

To improve overall stability in this pose, ensure the shoulder joint and scapula are stabilised. This can be achieved by activating the serratus anterior and rotator cuff muscles. To engage the serratus anterior, press into the ground with full force while externally rotating the hands. Additionally, the serratus anterior muscles help prevent winging of the scapula (where the scapula moves outward like wings, compromising stability).

Keep your fingers firmly engaged to protect your wrists. Expanding the fingers is also beneficial for most individuals as it increases the base of support.

Adho Mukha Vrksasana requires complete coordination between all major muscle groups, especially those of the trunk, including the trapezius, latissimus dorsi, spinal erectors, core, and quadratus lumborum.

The good news is that once learnt correctly, it will become significantly easier with practice.

Modifications

- **Progression (Variation):** If you wish to progress, you can try stretching additional muscles by interlacing your legs just like in Garduasana (Eagle Pose).
- **Regression (Wall Support):** Those who are unable to perform this pose correctly should opt for the wall-supported variation instead.
- **Prop Work:** You can perform this asana with yoga blocks for better stability.

Section IV
The Final Stretch

Frequently Asked Questions

Every yoga *sadhak* (practitioner) encounters various doubts relating to yoga. These doubts plague our minds until we get the right answers. However, more often than not, we keep these doubts in our subtle minds and never find time to clarify them. In this segment, we will explore all the common questions one may encounter.

Is yoga only about physical postures?

No, yoga has multiple limbs, of which asana is just one. In fact, yoga was initially focused on meditation and meditative asanas, with physical asanas introduced later. Based on documented evidence, more advanced asanas were added between 900–1300 CE.

Can anyone do yoga?

Almost anyone can practise yoga, regardless of caste, creed, gender, race, religion, or age. However, there are a few conditions when yoga should be avoided.

Is yoga suitable for children and teenagers?

Yes, yoga is well-suited for children and teenagers. The minimum age for children to practise yoga is 5-8 years. However, many yoga teachers suggest the 8-year mark, as this is when the alveoli sacs are sufficiently developed (Rehman and Bacha 2023).

How often should I practise yoga?

You can practise yoga every day, except for hot yoga. The physical form of yoga comes in various styles, most of which can be practised daily. However, if you practise an intense style of yoga, you may take a day off once a week. Practices such as pranayama, mudras, dhyana, dharana, and mantras can be practised daily.

Can yoga help with fat loss?

Yoga is evidence-backed for fat loss. All forms of hatha yoga are helpful in this regard. However, Vinyasa yoga is the best as it can help burn as many as 500–600 calories per hour. Believe it or not, it is difficult to burn that many calories with various other exercise regimes.

How long does a typical yoga session last?

Typically, a yoga session lasts about half an hour to an hour. The length of a yoga session may vary based on the style of yoga and the practitioner's intention.

What is the significance of 'Namaste' in yoga?

Namaste or Namaskar has three aspects: meaning, form (mudra), and intention.

- **Meaning:** The literal meaning of 'Namaste' is bowing down in respect. It is made up of two words: *Namah* = Bow down and *Te* = You.
- **Form (Mudra):** The Namaste is often accompanied by a specific mudra known as the 'Anjali Mudra' or 'Namaskar Mudra' (salutation gesture). This mudra is believed to enhance coordination between the two hemispheres of the brain.
- **Intention:** Namaskar is often greeted with the intention, 'I bow down to the divinity within you with the divinity within me'.

In conclusion, Namaste is a way to show gratitude to the *Brahman* (Cosmos).

Do I need to be in good shape to start yoga?

Not necessarily. Here, what we are referring to as yoga is mostly the physical form of yoga. According to most renowned yogis, asanas were invented to keep our bodies healthy and disease-free (*nirogi kaya*). Therefore, even if we are not in good shape, we can still practise yoga. However, I recommend a gradual approach to building the practice.

Can yoga help with stress and anxiety?

Yoga is evidence-backed in dealing with stress, anxiety, and similar conditions. Therefore, if you suffer from either of these, yoga can be a cost-effective solution. However, if you suffer from a chronic psychological condition, consult a qualified professional first.

Can yoga be a complete workout on its own?

Absolutely, yoga is a complete workout on its own. It offers multiple benefits that many other exercise regimes struggle to provide. However, if you are looking for muscle hypertrophy or aesthetic gains, progress may be slow unless you incorporate resistance training equipment with yoga.

What is the role of a yoga instructor?

The primary role of a yoga instructor is to guide their students/ clients towards their intent while ensuring safety. Instructors rely on cues and safe touches to do so. It may sound simple but can be tricky, as each student/client is unique with different intentions. Often, an instructor must counsel students towards the right path. Most yoga instructors also demonstrate asanas for enhanced clarity. At times, they may teach the science and philosophy of yoga.

How to wake up feeling fresh?

To wake up feeling fresh, the best approach is to manage the circadian rhythm correctly. The circadian rhythm is the biological clock of the human body, regulated primarily by the pineal gland, which secretes the hormone melatonin. The circadian rhythm depends on various physiological functions. Ideally, we should follow the solar and lunar cycle for regulating the biological clock. Moreover, avoid screens and lights at night, as the brain relies on blue light to distinguish between day and night. Sleeping early helps us wake up refreshed.

If someone is chronically sleep-deprived, the best course of action is to get 8–10 hours of sleep daily. It is worth noting that some individuals perform well with only six hours of sleep, while others need more. A consistent sleep-wake schedule is also crucial. Including an apple in breakfast is also beneficial as it contains natural sugar, which breaks down slowly, providing a constant supply of energy, which keeps us active throughout the day.

How to sleep well?

To sleep well, we must become more predictable for our bodies by maintaining certain constants, such as our sleep schedule, bed, and pillow. Practising yoga can also reinforce balanced nervous and endocrine systems, which, in turn, improve sleep quality. It is essential to avoid smoking and drinking alcohol. Forming better habits, avoiding caffeine at least four hours before sleep, and limiting dependence on caffeine can also help. Lastly, keeping the room as dark as possible is beneficial to calm both the brain and body.

Can cortisol affect my sleep pattern?

Cortisol is a critical hormone in the body, often referred to as the stress hormone. It is secreted by the adrenal glands and is a glucocorticoid hormone that influences metabolism, immune response, and inflammation. Hormones like cortisol can hinder our sleep-wake cycle. Cortisol levels should be optimal, rising in the morning and decreasing at night.

- **The vicious cycle of stress:** Typically, cortisol levels should decrease in the evening, while melatonin levels (the sleep hormone) increase. If this natural process is disrupted, it affects the brain's sleep signals, resulting in poor sleep quality, frequent waking, and light sleep. Chronic sleep deprivation leads to more stress, perpetuating the cycle.

To break this cycle, we can lower stress through various yoga practices, such as Yoga Nidra, restorative yoga, hatha yoga, and pranayama. Furthermore, establishing a sleep schedule, following a healthy diet, and adopting a healthy lifestyle are beneficial. In the case of chronic sleep deprivation, it is best to consult a doctor.

Can yoga improve cardio endurance?

Yes, yoga can greatly improve cardiovascular endurance. With cardiovascular diseases on the rise, experts suggest cardio practices to keep the heart and body healthy. In one study, yoga was found to perform better in some cardiorespiratory fitness parameters than aerobic activities (Sovová et al., 2015). For better results, practitioners should adopt healthy eating habits along with pranayama, asanas, mantras, and proper relaxation (shavasana).

Which yoga form is right for me?

There are various ways to practise hatha yoga, including Vinyasa, traditional hatha, Ashtanga Vinyasa, and yin yoga. If you are unsure, consult a yoga teacher. The correct form/style depends on factors such as age, intention, conditions/ailments, strength, flexibility, and previous experience.

Do I need to be flexible to do yoga?

No, you can practise yoga and gradually improve your flexibility, as it helps release tight muscles. The terms 'tightened muscles' and 'shortened muscles' are often used interchangeably. Muscles become tight due to prolonged stress and repetitive movements. Practising yoga helps to lengthen them, improving their range of motion. Additionally, yoga works on soft connective tissues like fascia, ligaments, tendons, and cartilage. Together, these mechanisms enhance flexibility. If you are already flexible, practising strength-oriented asanas is recommended.

Is yoga a religion?

Yoga is a way to live a healthy life, but it is not a religion. It comes with voluntary instructions, similar to a doctor's advice. Yoga discusses energies and their manifestations but does not involve authoritative figures. Essentially, yoga is a science meant for everyone. While some practices can be integrated with religion, they are not compulsory.

Do we need a spiritual belief to practise yoga?

No, spiritual belief is not necessary. Yoga has several limbs, each catering to different people. Various yogic limbs do not require spiritual beliefs, such as traditional hatha yoga, pranayama, several types of meditation, and mudras. However, there are limbs where spirituality does matter, such as mantra, Jnana yoga, and bhakti yoga. Practitioners can choose the type of practice that suits them best.

Is yoga research- or evidence-backed?

Yoga is, for the most part, science- or evidence-backed. In this book, I have cited studies wherever appropriate. I have personally read thousands of research articles on yoga and believe me when I say that yoga is indeed backed by science. I can assure you that at least hundreds of studies are likely ongoing as you read this. About 90 per cent of the yoga research I have encountered reports positive outcomes. However, it is important to note that research is an ongoing process. Some concepts of yoga that we cannot comprehend today may be understood in the future. Furthermore, the best thing about this practice is that it is interdisciplinary in nature, covering physiology, psychology, and neuroscience.

How can yoga benefit athletes and sports enthusiasts?

Most athletes and sports enthusiasts train for a specific sport. As we know, each sport has particular mechanisms and thus unique requirements. Moreover, every athlete has a unique body that adapts to training differently. However, regardless of the sport we play, some muscles can benefit greatly from yogic practice. For instance, athletes may find hamstring and calf muscle stretches particularly beneficial.

Does a gym enthusiast need yoga?

Resistance training, as commonly practised in gymnasiums, has various advantages. However, if performed incorrectly, it can cause imbalances, resulting in tendon stiffness (Kubo et al., 2007). Yoga can help alleviate these muscle imbalances. Moreover, yoga offers several other benefits that everyone, including gym enthusiasts, can greatly benefit from.

Is hot yoga better than other forms of yoga?

Hot yoga is not necessarily better than hatha, vinyasa, or Ashtanga Vinyasa in terms of burning calories, preventing injuries, improving flexibility, and other parameters. However, it does offer many of the same benefits as other yoga practices. Hot yoga is particularly popular in colder climates. Ultimately, if hot yoga resonates with you, you should practise it without worry, as there is still much to gain.

Can meditation improve my brain functioning?

There are various types of meditation, each with its own level of difficulty, point of focus, technique, and recruitment of brain regions. Despite these differences, meditation techniques have been shown to significantly affect brain function (Fox et al., 2014). Thus, practising meditation can be more beneficial than the time and effort it requires.

Why won't my brain stop thinking?

We experience about six thousand thoughts a day (Tseng and Poppenk 2020), which means we have several thoughts per minute. These thoughts are less noticeable when we are occupied with tasks. However, during meditation, we become more aware of them. Some of these thoughts may have a negative origin, and if we dwell on them, they may manifest as negative emotions. The way we deal with these thoughts varies across different yoga practices. I would suggest accepting these thoughts without being overly concerned by them.

How can I calm my mind?

To calm the mind, I believe yoga is one of the best cost-effective practices available. Yoga comprises various limbs, each working uniquely to bring serenity. For example, dirgha swasana (three-part breath), pranayama, yoga nidra, dharana (mindfulness, concentration, and visualisation), and dhyana (meditation and absorption) are all effective techniques.

Is it necessary to keep the eyes closed while practising meditation?

No, not necessarily. Yoga acknowledges that not everyone can meditate with their eyes closed. For this reason, some meditation styles involve gazing at mandalas, nature, temples, sculptures, deities, etc. However, most of these styles emphasise gazing at *sattvik* (virtuous) objects. The idea is to begin with external objects and gradually move towards internalisation. Over time, you may find it easier to meditate with your eyes closed.

How can I prevent falling asleep during a meditation class?

It is entirely normal for beginners to experience this. However, there are a few steps you can take to avoid it:

- Avoid meditating in a reclining position
- Avoid meditating on your bed
- Try musical mindfulness
- Ensure you get adequate sleep each day
- Practise meditation 2–4 hours after a meal
- Initially, try meditating with the curtains open or in a well-lit room
- Build your practice gradually, and it will become easier with time

What is Yoga therapy?

Yoga does have therapeutic applications. When these applications are used to treat medical conditions, it is often referred to as yoga therapy. Numerous studies are available on the therapeutic effects of Yoga, and it is frequently integrated into complementary and alternative medicine (CAM). However, I recommend only engaging in yoga therapy under the guidance of a qualified professional. It is essential to ensure that the professional is proficient in the therapeutic applications of yoga before proceeding.

Unmasking Popular Myths

Myth: Yoga is Only for Women

Fact: No, yoga can be practised by anyone. In fact, yoga is equally effective for everyone. However, some classes are specifically designed for women, such as pre- and post-natal yoga, and PCOS/PCOD sessions.

Myth: Flexibility Is Always Good

Fact: While loose ligaments are often associated with flexibility, there is always a risk of hypermobility. Hypermobility occurs when our joints have a greater range of motion than normal. For instance, some practitioners tend to hyperextend their knees in Ardha Uttanasana (Standing Half Forward Bend), which causes the joints to extend beyond their natural range. Hypermobility is linked with lax ligaments and can cause pain and discomfort (Saremi et al., 2016). Therefore, flexibility can come at a cost, and if you are hypermobile, it's advisable to practise muscle-strengthening asanas.

Myth: Yoga Advocates a Vegan Diet

Fact: People in the West often assume the yogic diet is strictly vegan. However, contrary to this belief, the traditional yogic diet includes milk-based products. Ancient yogic scriptures encourage the consumption of various dairy products. In India, the cow is considered sacred and is cared for like family. In many places, cows are protected until they die naturally. This practice, common in my native place, aligns with the principle of Ahimsa (non-violence), making milk products acceptable in the yogic diet.

Myth: Practising Strength-Based Yoga Can Hamper Children's Growth

Fact: No, strength-based practices can, in fact, improve overall growth. Children can safely practise strength-oriented asanas without concerns. The key is to ensure they follow proper form and injury prevention guidelines. Research shows that strength-based practices do not hinder bone growth in children (Malina, Robert M., 2006). Additionally, these practices offer benefits such as prehabilitation and improved bone density (Dahab K.S. and McCambridge T.M., 2009).

Myth: Neck and Spine Alignment Can Differ

Fact: A common misconception in the yoga community is that the neck and spine can be aligned differently. This is particularly evident in poses like forward bends, backbends, and trunk rotations. For example, in Bhujangasana (Cobra Pose), practitioners are often instructed to gaze upwards, which puts the neck in an uncomfortable position. The rest of the spine is in a gentle backbend, but the neck becomes overly extended. The neck is an inextricable part of the spine, and its alignment should ideally follow the rest of the spine's movement.

Myth: Bone Growth Can Occur After Puberty

Fact: Bones grow through growth plates, which fuse after puberty, meaning further growth is not possible. Some claim that poses like Tadasana (Palm Tree Pose) or Vrksasana (Tree Pose) can increase height. However, once growth plates have fused, yoga or any other non-invasive treatment will not promote further growth.

Myth: Fat Loss and Weight Loss Are the Same

Fact: Fat loss and weight loss are often used interchangeably, but they are not the same. Fat loss reduces the body's fat percentage, while weight loss can be due to various factors such as muscle atrophy, fluid loss, etc.

Myth: ***Raising the Arms Overhead Increases Blood Pressure***

Fact: No, it does not. Raising the arms is unlikely to elevate blood pressure. Our brain requires about 10-15% of our total blood supply, which is substantial. Therefore, if the heart is already accustomed to supplying blood to the brain, raising the arms is an easier task and does not typically cause an issue.

Myth: Osteoarthritis Only Affects the Knee Joint

Fact: This is a common misconception. Osteoarthritis can affect any moveable joint in the body, not just the knee.

Myth: Popping Joints Causes Osteoarthritis

Fact: The popping sound you hear in joints, known as crepitus, is generally harmless. Cracking joints like the knuckles does not cause osteoarthritis (Deweber K, et al., 2011). However, if the popping is accompanied by pain, it could indicate a problem. Crepitus is often the result of air build-up in the synovial fluid of a joint.

Myth: You Can Lose Fat from Specific Areas (Spot Reduction)

Fact: No, you cannot target fat loss from a specific part of your body. Fat distribution, such as on the face, belly, upper arms, or thighs, reflects your total body fat. Spot reduction, the idea of targeting fat loss in specific areas, is not supported by scientific studies.

Myth: 'No Pain, No Gain'

Fact: This misconception persists not only in yoga but in general fitness. Pain is not an indicator of progress. If you experience pain during yoga, it usually means you are not doing the pose correctly. It's important to differentiate between muscle fatigue and pain. Yoga follows the principle of 'Ahimsa' (non-violence), which also applies to your body—pushing yourself too hard can lead to injury.

Myth: Core-Centric Asanas Will Give You a Flat Belly

Fact: Core-centric asanas like Navasana (Boat Pose) are not specifically designed to give you a flat belly. Belly fat is a combination of subcutaneous and visceral fat. While core exercises improve posture and support the spine, they do not directly burn significant calories as spot reduction is not possible.

Myth: Yoga Is Merely a Static Stretch

Fact: Asanas are not just stretches. Yoga involves both contraction and stretching of muscles. Hatha yoga, in particular, is considered a form of resistance or strength training, with isometric contractions occurring in many poses.

Myth: More Sweating Means More Fat Loss

Fact: No, sweating is not an indicator of fat loss. Sweating is the body's mechanism to regulate temperature, and the amount of sweat can be influenced by factors like fat percentage, stress, external temperature, and genetics.

Myth: I Can Eat Unhealthy Food if I Practise Yoga

Fact: While occasional indulgence is fine, it's not advisable to rely on unhealthy food regularly. Yoga promotes a healthy lifestyle, including mindful eating. Consistently eating unhealthy food may counteract the benefits of your yoga practice.

Myth: All Calories Are the Same

Fact: Not all calories are the same. Foods may have equal calories but different nutritional values. The way each food interacts with your body varies depending on its nutrients.

Myth: Eating Less Equals Fat Loss

Fact: This is a complex misconception. Simply eating less does not guarantee fat loss. While maintaining a calorie deficit is key, metabolism plays a crucial role. Sudden calorie restriction can slow metabolism, hindering fat loss. It's better to reduce calorie intake gradually and combine it with muscle training and aerobic yoga practices.

BEYOND THE SCOPE OF YOGA

I believe yoga is for everyone and is certainly free from bias. However, there are instances where yoga is not suitable. My intention is not to discourage anyone but to set clear boundaries. In some cases, ayurveda, the sister science of yoga, may be helpful. Most of these considerations are intuitive, but occasionally a slight delay in addressing the matter can mean the difference between life and death for someone. Therefore, I will leave no stone unturned.

Acute Injuries

Acute injuries are more common in sports and very rare in yoga. However, I do not intend to rule out the possibility of such injuries occurring in a yoga class. These injuries typically happen in a split second. Examples include sudden twisting of the knees, falls, shoulder injuries, motor vehicle accidents, dislocations, and other wounds. In such cases, immediate medical intervention may be necessary. Yoga is not designed to treat acute injuries, although it can play an instrumental role in rehabilitation.

Diagnosis

Yoga does not address the diagnosis of any condition. Thus, it is essential to rely on conventional medical methods for diagnosis.

Chronic or Severe Conditions

There are chronic or severe conditions where beginning with only yoga is not ideal. In these cases, continuing with conventional treatments alongside yoga may be a more effective approach.

Infectious Diseases

Diseases that can spread by any means may fall outside the scope of yoga. For instance, tuberculosis, HIV, COVID-19, etc. If you are unwell, take precautions and stay indoors until the condition has been properly diagnosed.

Complications in Pregnancy

In the case of a complicated pregnancy, it is advisable to stick to conventional treatment options. However, if your doctor recommends yoga, you may continue practising it under their guidance.

Stones

If you have a cyst, stone, or any mineral deposit in an organ (kidney stones, gallstones, etc.), consulting a qualified doctor should be your priority. However, yoga can help manage pain and as a preventive measure.

Unidentified Condition

If you are experiencing symptoms of an unknown underlying condition, it is best to refrain from practising Yoga until the root cause has been identified.

In an Emergency

Yoga is not intended to address conditions that require immediate and urgent attention. In such cases, seek conventional treatments. For instance, heart attacks, strokes, severe allergic reactions, or other life-threatening situations. I encourage everyone to learn basic first aid and CPR.

Acknowledgements

I am profoundly grateful to my mother, brother, father, Bholi Parihar, Julie Parihar, Satyam Tiwari, and my extended family for believing in my vision and supporting me throughout the journey of this book. Without them, this book would not have been possible. I commend Bholi Parihar for modelling for the asanas, and if you admire the illustrations, you have Julie Parihar's artistic eye to thank. Initially, there was some uncertainty about her skills, but she surpassed all expectations with flying colours.

I am immensely grateful to the entire Hay House team for making an exception to publish a well-illustrated book. Special gratitude goes to Aditya Jarial, Sonali Pawar, Raghav Khattar, the design team, and everyone else at Hay House India for their patience and diligent work. At times, they undertook several reiterations to polish the book to its fullest.

I feel humbled by organisations such as Siddhi Yoga and Mindhouse for teaching me the value of discipline in life. I am sincerely indebted to my teachers for their quintessential role in guiding me towards wisdom, purpose, and spirituality. I am also grateful to those who considered reviewing the book: Ami Gantra, Dr Ishwar V. Basavaraddi, Dr Gourav Dwivedi, Vidhey Tirpude, and Satyam Tiwari.

Finally, I extend my heartfelt thanks to the key people who sparked creativity within me: Ashish and Varsha Ahuja, Acharya Kaushal Kumar, Manisha Aggarwal, Vijender Singh, Subham Khandelwal, Shubhendu Roy, Rahul Rawat, Brijesh Mishra, Ankit Singh, Mohit Dutt, and Atul Mishra.

Additionally, I am grateful to those who helped me discover another side of myself: Saurabh Mishra, Karan Singh, Neha Sharma, Amrita Tomar, Sumit Sharma, Rajesh Watts, Sarita Sharma, Nishtha and Jitesh Gandhi, Ashay Gupta, Anuradha Sabharwal, Kiran Ghosh, Lavina Rastogi, Geeta Singh, Nazia Parwin, Charu Phutela, Kartik Gupta, Abhishek Bharti Gopal, Meena Prajapati, Mohit Khurana, Gulshan Pandey, Naveen Poudel, Master Arya, Pawan Negi, Preetam Mata, Sandeep Solanki, Ashish Prashad, Gaurav Negi, Ravi Kumar, Gaurav Dhande, Shrija Pandey, Vikas Bamel, Divya Aggarwal, and Kuldeep Parmar.

I am grateful to everyone who stood by my side and helped me gain new perspectives on life. I love connecting with you all.

Bibliography

Agre, Sharayu, Ronika Agrawal, and Sayed Ishrat Fatima Asgar. 'Effect of Suryanamaskar on Stress Levels in SSC Students.' *Indian Journal of Public Health Research & Development* 12, no. 3 (2021): 218–23. https://doi.org/10.37506/ijphrd.v12i3.16151.

Arora, S., and J. Bhattacharjee. 'Modulation of Immune Responses in Stress by Yoga.' *International Journal of Yoga* 1, no. 2 (July 2008): 45-55. https://doi.org/10.4103/0973-6131.43541.

Carroll, J., A. Blansit, R. M. Otto, and J. W. Wygand. 'The Metabolic Requirements of Vinyasa Yoga.' *Medicine & Science in Sports & Exercise* 35, no. 5 (2003): S155.

Chanavirut, Raoyrin, et al. 'Yoga Exercise Increases Chest Wall Expansion and Lung Volumes in Young Healthy Thais.' *Thai J Physiol Sci* 19, no. 1 (2006): 1-7.

Cherpak, Colleen E. 'Mindful Eating: A Review of How the Stress-Digestion-Mindfulness Triad May Modulate and Improve Gastrointestinal and Digestive Function.' *Integrative Medicine (Encinitas)* 18, no. 4 (August 2019): 48-53.

Chin, Michael S., and Stefanos N. Kales. 'Understanding Mind–Body Disciplines: A Pilot Study of Paced Breathing and Dynamic Muscle Contraction on Autonomic Nervous System Reactivity.' *Stress and Health* 35, no. 4 (2019): 542-548.

Colligan, Thomas W., and Eileen M. Higgins. 'Workplace Stress.' *Journal of Workplace Behavioral Health* 21, no. 2 (2006): 89-97. https://doi.org/10.1300/J490v21n02_07.

Connor, R. C. 'Dolphin Social Intelligence: Complex Alliance Relationships in Bottlenose Dolphins and a Consideration of Selective Environments for Extreme Brain Size Evolution in Mammals.' *Philosophical Transactions of the Royal Society B: Biological Sciences*

362, no. 1480 (April 29, 2007): 587–602. https://doi.org/10.1098/rstb.2006.1997.

Cramer, Holger, et al. 'A Systematic Review and Meta-Analysis of Yoga for Low Back Pain.' *The Clinical Journal of Pain* 29, no. 5 (2013): 450–60. https://doi.org/10.1097/AJP.0b013e3182546f0c.

Cramer, Holger, et al. 'Effects of Yoga on Cardiovascular Disease Risk Factors: A Systematic Review and Meta-Analysis.' *International Journal of Cardiology* 173, no. 2 (2014): 170–83. https://doi.org/10.1016/j.ijcard.2014.03.073.

Dahab, Katherine S., and Todd M. McCambridge. 'Strength Training in Children and Adolescents: Raising the Bar for Young Athletes?' *Sports Health* 1, no. 3 (May 2009): 223-226. https://doi.org/10.1177/1941738109334215.

Deepeshwar, Singh, et al. 'Effect of Yoga-Based Lifestyle Intervention on Patients with Knee Osteoarthritis: A Randomized Controlled Trial.' *Frontiers in Psychiatry* 9 (2018): 180. https://doi.org/10.3389/fpsyt.2018.00180.

Deweber, Kevin, Matthew Olszewski, and Robert Ortolano. 'Knuckle Cracking and Hand Osteoarthritis.' *Journal of the American Board of Family Medicine* 24, no. 2 (March-April 2011): 169-174. https://doi.org/10.3122/jabfm.2011.02.100156.

Dhar, N., S. Chaturvedi, and D. Nandan. 'Spiritual Health Scale 2011: Defining and Measuring Four Dimensions of Health.' *Indian Journal of Community Medicine* 36, no. 4 (October 2011): 275–82. https://doi.org/10.4103/0970-0218.91329.

Falkenberg, R. I., C. Eising, and M. L. Peters. 'Yoga and Immune System Functioning: A Systematic Review of Randomized Controlled Trials.' *Journal of Behavioral Medicine* 41 (2018): 467-482.

Falkenberg, R. I., C. Eising, and M. L. Peters. 'Yoga and Immune System Functioning: A Systematic Review of Randomized Controlled Trials.' *Journal of Behavioral Medicine* 41, no. 4 (2018): 467–82. https://doi.org/10.1007/s10865-018-9914-y.

Fernández-Rodríguez, Rubén, et al. 'Effectiveness of Pilates and Yoga to Improve Bone Density in Adult Women: A Systematic Review and Meta-Analysis.' *PloS One* 16, no. 5 (2021): e0251391. https://doi.org/10.1371/journal.pone.0251391.

Fox, Kieran C. R., Jared M. Nijeboer, Jason Dixon, and Kalina Christoff. 'Is Meditation Associated with Altered Brain Structure? A Systematic Review and Meta-Analysis of Morphometric Neuroimaging in Meditation Practitioners.' *Neuroscience & Biobehavioral Reviews* 43 (2014): 48-73.

Ganesh, HR Shree, Pailoor Subramanya, and Vivek Udupa. 'Role of Yoga Therapy in Improving Digestive Health and Quality of Sleep in an Elderly Population: A Randomized Controlled Trial.' *Journal of Bodywork and Movement Therapies* 27 (2021): 692-697.

Gautam, S., R. Kumar, U. Kumar, et al. 'Yoga Maintains Th17/Treg Cell Homeostasis and Reduces the Rate of T Cell Aging in Rheumatoid Arthritis: A Randomized Controlled Trial.' *Scientific Reports* 13 (2023): 14924. https://doi.org/10.1038/s41598-023-42231-w.

Golec de Zavala, Agnieszka, Dorottya Lantos, and Deborah Bowden. 'Yoga Poses Increase Subjective Energy and State Self-Esteem in Comparison to 'Power Poses.'' *Frontiers in Psychology* 8 (2017): 752. https://doi.org/10.3389/fpsyg.2017.00752.

Gordon, Julianne. *The Metabolic Demand of a Vinyasa Yoga Session.* PhD diss., University of Saskatchewan, 2014.

Gothe, Neha P., and Edward McAuley. 'Yoga Is as Good as Stretching–Strengthening Exercises in Improving Functional Fitness Outcomes: Results from a Randomized Controlled Trial.' *Journals of Gerontology Series A: Biomedical Sciences and Medical Sciences* 71, no. 3 (2016): 406-411.

Gothe, Neha P., and Edward McAuley. 'Yoga Is as Good as Stretching–Strengthening Exercises in Improving Functional Fitness Outcomes: Results From a Randomized Controlled Trial.' *The Journals of Gerontology: Series A* 71, no. 3 (March 2016): 406–411. https://doi.org/10.1093/gerona/glv127.

Gothe, Neha P., I. Khan, J. Hayes, E. Erlenbach, and J. S. Damoiseaux. 'Yoga Effects on Brain Health: A Systematic Review of the Current Literature.' *Brain Plasticity* 5, no. 1 (2019): 105–22. https://doi.org/10.3233/BPL-190084.

Govindaraj, R., S. Karmani, S. Varambally, and B. N. Gangadhar. 'Yoga and Physical Exercise—A Review and Comparison.' *International Review of Psychiatry* 28, no. 3 (2016): 242–53. https://doi.org/10.3109/09540261.2016.1160878.

Grabara, Małgorzata. 'Effects of Hatha Yoga Exercises on Spine Flexibility in Young Adults.' *Biomedical Human Kinetics* 8, no. 1 (2016): 113–16. https://doi.org/10.1515/bhk-2016-0016.

Graubard, R., A. Perez-Sanchez, and R. Katta. 'Stress and Skin: An Overview of Mind-Body Therapies as a Treatment Strategy in Dermatology.' *Dermatology Practical & Conceptual* 11, no. 4 (2021): e2021091. https://doi.org/10.5826/dpc.1104a91.

Guidotti, Roberto, Claudia Del Gratta, Maria Grazia Perrucci, Gian Luca Romani, and Antonino Raffone. 'Neuroplasticity Within and Between Functional Brain Networks in Mental Training Based on Long-Term Meditation.' *Brain Sciences* 11, no. 8 (2021): 1086. https://doi.org/10.3390/brainsci11081086.

Ha, Ju-Young, and Seon-Hwa Ban. 'Effects of Mind–Body Programs on Infertile Women: A Systematic Review and Meta-Analysis of Randomized Controlled Trials.' *Asian Nursing Research* 15, no. 2 (2021): 77–88. https://doi.org/10.1016/j.anr.2021.01.002.

Hagins, Marshall, Terry Selfe, and Kim Innes. 'Effectiveness of Yoga for Hypertension: Systematic Review and Meta-Analysis.' *Evidence-Based Complementary and Alternative Medicine* 2013 (2013). https://doi.org/10.1155/2013/649836.

Hartfiel, Nicholas, Catherine Burton, Jacqueline Rycroft-Malone, Graeme Clarke, Jonathan Havenhand, Sat Bir S. Khalsa, and Rhiannon T. Edwards. 'Yoga for Reducing Perceived Stress and Back Pain at Work.' *Occupational Medicine* 62, no. 8 (December 2012): 606-612. https://doi.org/10.1093/occmed/kqs168.

Hoge, Elizabeth A., Sarah J. Bui, Naomi M. Palitz, Brandon M. Schwarz, John W. Pollack, Jonathan Greenberg, Cameron S. Anderson, Eric B. Loucks, and Michelle G. Craske. 'Mindfulness-Based Stress Reduction vs Escitalopram for the Treatment of Adults with Anxiety Disorders: A Randomized Clinical Trial.' *JAMA Psychiatry* 80, no. 1 (2023): 13-21.

Hong, A. R., and S. W. Kim. 'Effects of Resistance Exercise on Bone Health.' *Endocrinology and Metabolism (Seoul)* 33, no. 4 (2018): 435-444. https://doi.org/10.3803/EnM.2018.33.4.435.

Jayasinghe, Satyajit R. 'Yoga in Cardiac Health (A Review).' *European Journal of Preventive Cardiology* 11, no. 5 (2004): 369–75. https://doi.org/10.1097/01.hjr.0000138318.43811.10.

Joshua, S., and C. Dunbar. 'Cardiovascular and Metabolic Responses to Vinyasa Yoga and Paced Surya Namaskar B.' *Journal of Yoga & Physical Therapy* 6, no. 2 (2016): 230.

Kan, Laidi, et al. 'The Effects of Yoga on Pain, Mobility, and Quality of Life in Patients with Knee Osteoarthritis: A Systematic Review.' *Evidence-Based Complementary and Alternative Medicine* (2016). https://doi.org/10.1155/2016/6016532.

Kannan, Priya, et al. 'Yoga and Pilates Compared to Pelvic Floor Muscle Training for Urinary Incontinence in Elderly Women: A Randomised Controlled Pilot Trial.' *Complementary Therapies in Clinical Practice* 46 (2022): 101502. https://doi.org/10.1016/j.ctcp.2022.101502.

Kubo, Keitaro, Hiroaki Morimoto, Hidetaka Komuro, Narihiko Yata, Shinichi Tsunoda, Hisashi Kanehisa, and Tetsuo Fukunaga. 'Effects of Plyometric and Weight Training on Muscle-Tendon Complex and Jump Performance.' *Medicine & Science in Sports & Exercise* 39, no. 10 (2007): 1801-1810.

Kumar, A., R. C. Kapse, N. Paul, A. M. Vanjare, and S. N. Omkar. 'Musculoskeletal Modeling and Analysis of Trikonasana.' *International Journal of Yoga* 11, no. 3 (September-December 2018): 201–207. https://doi.org/10.4103/ijoy.IJOY_1_18.

Kuppusamy, Maheshkumar, et al. 'Effects of Yoga Breathing Practice on Heart Rate Variability in Healthy Adolescents: A Randomized Controlled Trial.' *Integrative Medicine Research* 9, no. 1 (2020): 28–32. https://doi.org/10.1016/j.imr.2020.01.004.

Lu, Y. H., B. Rosner, G. Chang, and L. M. Fishman. 'Twelve-Minute Daily Yoga Regimen Reverses Osteoporotic Bone Loss.' *Topics in Geriatric Rehabilitation* 32, no. 2 (2016): 81-87. https://doi.org/10.1097/TGR.0000000000000085.

Madhivanan, Purnima, Karl Krupp, Renee Waechter, Rahul Shidhaye. 'Yoga for Healthy Aging: Science or Hype?' *Advances in Geriatric Medicine and Research* 3, no. 3 (July 2021): e210016. https://doi.org/10.20900/agmr20210016.

Maior, Alex Souto, and Marco Leandro Martins de Assis. 'Neuromuscular and Functional Responses Among Males Trained with Free Weights vs. Machines: Implications for Injury Prevention.' *International Journal of Strength and Conditioning* 3, no. 1 (2023).

Malina, Robert M. 'Weight Training in Youth: Growth, Maturation, and Safety: An Evidence-Based Review.' *Clinical Journal of Sport Medicine* 16, no. 6 (2006): 478-487.

Mohanty, Soubhagyalaxmi, Balaram Pradhan, and R. Nagathna. 'The Effect of Yoga Practice on Proprioception in Congenitally Blind Students.' *British Journal of Visual Impairment* 32, no. 2 (2014): 124-135.

Nishimune, Hiroshi, John A. Stanford, and Yasuo Mori. 'Role of Exercise in Maintaining the Integrity of the Neuromuscular Junction.' *Muscle & Nerve* 49, no. 3 (2014): 315–24. https://doi.org/10.1002/mus.24006.

Oates, Jennifer. 'The Effect of Yoga on Menstrual Disorders: A Systematic Review.' *The Journal of Alternative and Complementary Medicine* 23, no. 6 (2017): 407–17.

Pandey, Rajendra Kumar, A. Pande, and R. Joshi. 'Effects of 6 Months Yoga Program on Renal Functions and Quality of Life in Patients

Suffering from Chronic Kidney Disease.' *International Journal of Yoga* 10, no. 1 (2017): 3–8.

Paramasivam, Alagumariappan, et al. 'Analysis of Influence of Yoga-Asana on the Digestive Process Using Electrogastrograms.' In *Proceedings of the International Conference on Computing and Communication Systems: I3CS 2020, NEHU, Shillong, India*, 433–40. Singapore: Springer, 2021. https://doi.org/10.1007/978-981-16-1029-3_41.

Pascoe, Michaela C., and Isabelle E. Bauer. 'A Systematic Review of Randomised Control Trials on the Effects of Yoga on Stress Measures and Mood.' *Journal of Psychiatric Research* 68 (2015): 270-282.

Petric, Maja, Renata Vauhnik, and M. Jakovljevic. 'The Impact of Hatha Yoga Practice on Flexibility: A Pilot Study.' *Altern Integr Med* 3, no. 2 (2014): 2-10.

Polsgrove, M. Jay, Brandon M. Eggleston, and Roch J. Lockyer. 'Impact of 10-Weeks of Yoga Practice on Flexibility and Balance of College Athletes.' *International Journal of Yoga* 9, no. 1 (2016): 27–34. https://doi.org/10.4103/0973-6131.171710.

Ramlau-Hansen, C. H., et al. 'Is Smoking a Risk Factor for Decreased Semen Quality? A Cross-Sectional Analysis.' *Human Reproduction* 22, no. 1 (2007): 188–96. https://doi.org/10.1093/humrep/del364.

Rehman, S., and D. Bacha. 'Embryology, Pulmonary.' Last modified August 14, 2023. In *StatPearls* [Internet]. Treasure Island, FL: StatPearls Publishing, 2023-. https://www.ncbi.nlm.nih.gov/books/NBK544372/.

Ripoll, Elvira, and Darrell Mahowald. 'Hatha Yoga Therapy Management of Urologic Disorders.' *World Journal of Urology* 20 (2002): 306-309. https://doi.org/10.1007/s00345-002-0296-x.

Robertson, Claire J., Michael Hurley, and Fiona Jones. 'People's Beliefs About the Meaning of Crepitus in Patellofemoral Pain and the Impact of These Beliefs on Their Behaviour: A Qualitative Study.' *Musculoskeletal Science and Practice* 28 (2017): 59-64.

Ross, Alyson, et al. 'A Different Weight Loss Experience: A Qualitative Study Exploring the Behavioral, Physical, and Psychosocial Changes Associated with Yoga That Promote Weight Loss.' *Evidence-Based Complementary and Alternative Medicine* 2016 (2016). https://doi.org/10.1155/2016/2914742.

Saremi, H., A. Yavarikia, and N. Jafari. 'Generalized Ligamentous Laxity: An Important Predisposing Factor for Shoulder Injuries in Athletes.' *Iranian Red Crescent Medical Journal* 18, no. 6 (2016): e38903. https://doi.org/10.5812/ircmj.38903.

Sartori, D. V. B., P. R. Kawano, H. A. Yamamoto, R. Guerra, P. R. Pajolli, and J. L. Amaro. 'Pelvic Floor Muscle Strength Is Correlated with Sexual Function.' *Investigative and Clinical Urology* 62, no. 1 (2021): 79–84. https://doi.org/10.4111/icu.20190248.

Sengupta, P. 'Environmental and Occupational Exposure of Metals and Their Role in Male Reproductive Functions.' *Drug and Chemical Toxicology* 36, no. 3 (2013): 353–68. https://doi.org/10.3109/01480545.2012.710631.

Sengupta, P., P. Chaudhuri, and K. Bhattacharya. 'Male Reproductive Health and Yoga.' *International Journal of Yoga* 6, no. 2 (2013): 87–95. https://doi.org/10.4103/0973-6131.113391.

Sengupta, Pranab. 'Challenge of Infertility: How Protective the Yoga Therapy Is?' *Ancient Science of Life* 32, no. 1 (July 2012): 61-62. https://doi.org/10.4103/0257-7941.113796.

Singphow, C., S. Purohit, P. Tekur, S. Bista, S. N. Panigrahy, N. Raghuram, and H. R. Nagendra. 'Effect of Yoga on Stress, Anxiety, Depression, and Spinal Mobility in Computer Users with Chronic Low Back Pain.' *International Journal of Yoga* 15, no. 2 (2022): 114-121. https://doi.org/10.4103/ijoy.ijoy_9_22.

Solakoglu, O., B. D. Karatekin, Y. Yumusakhuylu, E. Mesci, and A. Icagasioglu. 'The Effect of Yoga Asana "Vrksasana (Tree Pose)" on Balance in Patients With Postmenopausal Osteoporosis: A Randomized Controlled Trial.' *American Journal of Physical Medicine & Rehabilitation* 101, no. 3 (2022): 255-261.

Sovová, E., V. Čajka, D. Pastucha, J. Malinčíková, L. Radová, and M. Sovová. 'Positive Effect of Yoga on Cardiorespiratory Fitness: A Pilot Study.' *International Journal of Yoga* 8, no. 2 (July-December 2015): 134-138. https://doi.org/10.4103/0973-6131.158482.

Sweta, K. M., Amruta Godbole, Hema H. Awasthi, and Uma Pandey. 'Effect of Mula Bandha Yoga in Mild Grade Pelvic Organ Prolapse: A Randomized Controlled Trial.' *International Journal of Yoga* 11, no. 2 (May-August 2018): 116-121. https://doi.org/10.4103/ijoy.IJOY_32_17.

Telles, Satyananda, and Nidhi Singh. 'Is Yoga a Suitable Treatment for Rheumatoid Arthritis: Current Opinion.' *Open Access Journal of Sports Medicine* 3 (2012): 81–87. https://doi.org/10.2147/OAJSM.S25707.

Thakur, Deepshikha, Subodh Saurabh Singh, and Mala Tripathi. 'Effect of Yoga on Polycystic Ovarian Syndrome: A Systematic Review.' *Journal of Bodywork and Movement Therapies* 27 (2021): 281–86. https://doi.org/10.1016/j.jbmt.2021.03.014.

Thirthalli, J., et al. 'Cortisol and Antidepressant Effects of Yoga.' *Indian Journal of Psychiatry* 55, Suppl. 3 (2013): S405–8. https://doi.org/10.4103/0019-5545.105556.

Tolahunase, M. R., Rajesh Sagar, Mohammad Faiq, and Ripudaman D. Dada. 'Yoga- and Meditation-Based Lifestyle Intervention Increases Neuroplasticity and Reduces the Severity of Major Depressive Disorder: A Randomized Controlled Trial.' *Restorative Neurology and Neuroscience* 36, no. 3 (2018): 423-442. https://doi.org/10.3233/RNN-170810.

Tolahunase, M., R. Sagar, and R. Dada. 'Impact of Yoga and Meditation on Cellular Aging in Apparently Healthy Individuals: A Prospective, Open-Label Single-Arm Exploratory Study.' *Oxidative Medicine and Cellular Longevity* (2017): 7928981. https://doi.org/10.1155/2017/7928981.

Tran, M. D., et al. 'Effects of Hatha Yoga Practice on the Health-Related Aspects of Physical Fitness.' *Preventive Cardiology* 4, no. 4 (2001): 165–70.

Tseng, Jean, and Jordan Poppenk. 'Brain Meta-State Transitions Demarcate Thoughts Across Task Contexts Exposing the Mental Noise of Trait Neuroticism.' *Nature Communications* 11 (2020): 3480. https://doi.org/10.1038/s41467-020-17255-9.

Verdam, Froukje J., et al. 'Human Intestinal Microbiota Composition Is Associated with Local and Systemic Inflammation in Obesity.' *Obesity* 21, no. 12 (2013): E607–15. https://doi.org/10.1002/oby.20466.